Absolute Beginner's Guide

to

WITHDRAWN

Alternative Medicine

Karen Lee Fontaine
with Bill Kaszubski

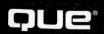

800 East 96th Street,
Indianapolis, Indiana 46240

Absolute Beginner's Guide to Alternative Medicine

Copyright © 2004 by Que Publishing

International Standard Book Number: 0-7897-3119-3

Library of Congress Catalog Card Number: 2004100876

Printed in the United States of America

First Printing: April 2004

07   06   05   7   6   5   4   3

Trademarks

All terms mentioned in this book that are known to be trademarks or service marks have been appropriately capitalized. Que Publishing cannot attest to the accuracy of this information. Use of a term in this book should not be regarded as affecting the validity of any trademark or service mark.

Warning and Disclaimer

Every effort has been made to make this book as complete and as accurate as possible, but no warranty or fitness is implied. The information provided is on an "as is" basis. The authors and the publisher shall have neither liability nor responsibility to any person or entity with respect to any loss or damages arising from the information contained in this book.

The content of this book is derived from *Healing Practices — Alternative Therapies for Nursing*, by Karen L. Fontaine, published by Prentice Hall: ISBN 0838503853.

Bulk Sales

Que Publishing offers excellent discounts on this book when ordered in quantity for bulk purchases or special sales. For more information, please contact

U.S. Corporate and Government Sales
1-800-382-3419
corpsales@pearsontechgroup.com

For sales outside of the U.S., please contact

International Sales
international@pearsoned.com

Executive Editor
Candace Hall

Acquisitions Editor
Karen Whitehouse

Development Editors
Bill Kaszubski
Karen Whitehouse

Managing Editor
Charlotte Clapp

Project Editor
Elizabeth Finney

Copy Editor
Karen Whitehouse

Indexer
Ken Johnson

Proofreader
Benjamin Berg

Publishing Coordinator
Sharry Lee Gregory

Interior Designer
Anne Jones

Cover Designer
Dan Armstrong

Page Layout
Eric S. Miller

Graphics
Laura Robbins

Contents at a Glance

Table of Contents

About the Authors

Karen Lee Fontaine is a nursing professor at Purdue University, the Calumet campus. She has authored many nursing books on topics such as mental health and psychiatric nursing. **Bill Kaszubski** lives in Los Angeles, where he writes about science, art, and technology.

We Want to Hear from You!

As the reader of this book, *you* are our most important critic and commentator. We value your opinion and want to know what we're doing right, what we could do better, what areas you'd like to see us publish in, and any other words of wisdom you're willing to pass our way.

As an executive editor for Que Publishing, I welcome your comments. You can email or write me directly to let me know what you did or didn't like about this book—as well as what we can do to make our books better.

Please note that I cannot help you with technical problems related to the topic of this book. We do have a User Services group, however, where I will forward specific technical questions related to the book.

When you write, please be sure to include this book's title and author as well as your name, email address, and phone number. I will carefully review your comments and share them with the author and editors who worked on the book.

Email   feedback@quepublishing.com

Mail: Candace Hall
           Executive Editor
           Que Publishing
           800 East 96th Street
           Indianapolis, IN 46240 USA

For more information about this book or another Que Publishing title, visit our Web site at www.quepublishing.com. Type the ISBN (excluding hyphens), or type in the title of a book in the Search field.

PART i

An Introduction to Alternative Medicine

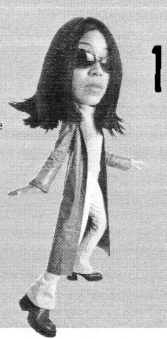

1

WHAT IS ALTERNATIVE MEDICINE ALL ABOUT?

According to a random survey conducted in 1997, 42% of Americans sought out and used one or more types of medical interventions that were not taught in medical schools and were not generally available in U.S. hospitals. This represented an eight percentage point increase over the 1990 results of the same survey. While the vast majority (96%) of these people were also seeking conventional treatment for their health problems, less than 40% of these people told their conventional doctors what they were doing. Clearly, something's going on with alternative medicine.

More than half of these Americans paid for the entire cost of treatment themselves, contributing to the estimated $27 billion spent on alternative medicine treatments in 1997—almost equal to U.S. consumers' out-of-pocket expenses for conventional physician's services in the same time period. In total, Americans made 629 million visits to alternative healers in 1997, nearly 243 million more visits than to all U.S. primary care physicians. While no comparable survey results have been published since then, all indications are that Americans have continued to embrace alternative therapies, most likely at an accelerating rate. Clearly, alternative medicine is a big business.

The mainstream medical community can no longer ignore alternative therapies. The public interest is extensive and growing. You have only to look at the proliferation of popular health books, health food stores, and clinics offering healing therapies to realize that this interest cannot be dismissed. In other words, Americans want something more than biomedicine, and they are willing to pay for it.

Why Are People Turning to Alternative Medicine?

Some people have the same goal for both conventional and alternative medicine, such as the use of both pain medications and acupuncture to control chronic pain. Others may have a different expectation for each approach: For example, seeing a conventional practitioner for antibiotics to eradicate an infection, and then using an alternative practitioner to improve natural immunity through a healthy lifestyle. Someone receiving chemotherapy may use meditation and visualization to control the side effects of the chemotherapeutic agents. People who combine conventional and alternative therapies are making therapeutic choices on their own and assuming responsibility for their own health (see Table 1.1).

Table 1.1   Thirteen Top Reasons People Seek Alternative Therapies, 1990–1997

Problem	Percentage of Sufferers
Neck problems	57
Back problems	48
Anxiety	43
Depression	41
Headaches	32
Arthritis	27
GI problems	27
Fatigue	27
Insomnia	26

Problem	Percentage of Sufferers
Sprain/strains	24
Allergies	17
Lung problems	13
Hypertension	12

Because alternative therapists are rushing to meet the demand, it is increasingly difficult for consumers to figure out how and where to get the best health care. It may be difficult to find reliable information to help separate the healers from those who pretend to have medical knowledge. You should beware of healers who display these characteristics:

- Say they have all the answers.
- Maintain that their therapy is the only effective therapy.
- Promise overnight success.
- Refuse to include other practitioners as part of the healing team.
- Seem more interested in money than in your well-being.

Some alternative specialties are more regulated and licensed than others, but none come with guarantees—any more than conventional medicine comes with guarantees. Many people locate alternative therapists through friends, family, an exercise instructor, health food stores, or referral lines at local hospitals. Most people don't speak with their conventional medicine providers about their use of alternative therapies, out of fear of embarrassment, ridicule, or discouragement. These fears are unreasonable. If your physician is judgmental and not pleased to see you taking an active interest in your health, then you may want to consider finding another physician. On the other hand, there's no doubt that your doctor knows more about medicine than you do (unless you're a doctor too!). By having an open and frank discussion, you can find therapies that help address your concerns while steering clear of those that are dangerous or hoaxes.

REASONS WHY PEOPLE CHOOSE ALTERNATIVE THERAPIES
- To pursue therapeutic benefit.
- To seek a degree of wellness not supported in biomedicine.
- To attend to quality-of-life issues.
- They prefer high personal involvement in decision-making.

continues

■ They believe conventional medicine treats symptoms, not underlying cause.

■ They find conventional medical treatments to be lacking or ineffective.

■ To avoid toxicities and/or invasiveness of conventional interventions.

■ To decrease use of prescribed or over-the-counter (OTC) medications.

■ To identify with a particular healing system as a part of cultural background.

What We Talk About When We Talk About Health

One of the first problems a healthcare consumer encounters when considering some type of non-traditional medical treatment is that of language. Many people regard the term "alternative medicine" as too narrow or misleading and are concerned that the term does not encompass a full understanding of traditional healing practices. It would be more helpful for a common language to be developed without people being captive to it. For consistency's sake, this guide will use the terms *conventional medicine* or *biomedicine* to describe standard Western medical practices and the terms *alternative medicine* or *complementary medicine* to describe the other healing practices that are this guide's focus.

However, there are no universally accepted terms. For example, the term alternative medicine is used more in the United States while complementary medicine is used in Europe, but do they really mean the same thing? And, should Western medicine be called Western medicine when it's practiced in the modern hospitals of India and Singapore? Confusion over the very terms used lies at the heart of much of the confusion about alternative medicine as a whole, especially as more and more information, often contradictory, becomes available to the consumer (see Table 1.2). Hopefully, this guide will help you organize and evaluate the information you have and discover, and allow you to make informed and considered decisions about your approach to maintaining and enhancing your health.

Table 1.2   Terms Used to Compare the Two Types of Medicine

Mainstream Medicine	Complementary/Alternative
Modern	Ancient
Western	Eastern
Allopathic	Homeopathic
Conventional	Unconventional
Orthodox	Traditional
Biomedicine	Natural medicine
Scientific	Indigenous healing methods

The line between conventional and alternative medicine is imprecise and frequently changing. For example, is the use of megavitamins or diet regimes to treat disease considered medicine, a lifestyle change, or both? Can having your pain lessened by massage be considered a medical therapy? How should spiritual healing and prayer—some of the oldest, most widely used, and least studied traditional approaches—be classified? Although the terms alternative or complementary are frequently used, in some instances they represent the primary treatment for an individual. Thus, conventional medicine sometimes assumes a secondary role and actually becomes a complement to the primary treatment plan.

Conventional Medicine

Conventional Western medicine is only about 200 years old. It is founded on the philosophical beliefs of René Descartes (1596–1650), who regarded the mind and body as separate, and on Sir Isaac Newton's (1642–1727) principles of physics, which view the universe as a large mechanical clock where everything operates in a linear, sequential form. This mechanistic perspective of medicine views the human body as a series of body parts. It also is a "reductionist" approach in which the person is converted into increasingly smaller components: systems, organs, cells, and biochemicals. Taking that idea further, people are reduced to patients, patients are reduced to bodies, and bodies are reduced to machines. Health is viewed as the absence of disease—in other words, nothing broken at the present time. The focus of sick care is on the symptoms of dysfunction. Doctors are trained to fix or repair broken parts through the use of drugs, radiation, surgery, or replacement of body parts. This approach is aggressive and militant, with physicians in a war against disease, and a take-no-prisoners attitude. Both consumers and practitioners of biomedicine believe it is better to do something rather than wait and see whether the body's natural processes resolve the problem, and attack the disease directly by medication or surgery rather than try to build up the person's resistance and ability to overcome the disease.

Biomedicine views the person primarily as a physical body, with the mind and spirit being separate and secondary, or at times, even irrelevant. It is powerful medicine in that it has virtually eliminated some infectious diseases such as smallpox and polio. As a "rescue" medicine, the biomedical approach is wonderful. It is highly effective in emergencies, traumatic injuries, bacterial infections, and some highly sophisticated surgeries. In these cases, treatment is fast, aggressive, and goal-oriented, with the responsibility for cure falling on the practitioner. The priority of intervention is on opposing and suppressing the symptoms of illness. This mindset can be seen in many medications with countering prefixes such as "an" or "anti"—analgesics, anesthetics, anti-inflammatories, antipyretics, and so on. Because conventional medicine is preoccupied with parts and symptoms and not with whole working systems of matter, energy, thoughts, and feelings, it doesn't do well with long-term systemic illnesses such as arthritis, heart disease, and hypertension.

Alternative Medicine

Alternative medicine is an umbrella term for hundreds of therapies drawn from all over the world. Many forms are based on the medical systems of older cultures, including Egyptian, Chinese, Asian Indian, Greek, and Native American, and have been handed down over thousands of years, both orally and as written records. Other therapies, such as osteopathy and naturopathy, have evolved in the United States over the past two centuries. Still others, such as some of the mind-body and bioelectromagnetic approaches, are on the frontier of scientific knowledge and understanding.

Although they represent diverse approaches, alternative therapies share certain attributes. They are based on the paradigm of whole systems, and the belief that people are more than physical bodies with fixable and replaceable parts. Mental, emotional, and spiritual components of well-being are considered to play a crucial and equal role in a person's state of health. Since body, mind, and spirit are one unified reality, illness is considered to affect, and be affected by, both body and mind. Even Hippocrates, the father of Western medicine, espoused a holistic orientation when he taught doctors to observe their patients' life circumstances and emotional states. Socrates agreed, declaring, "Curing the soul; that is the first thing." In alternative medicine, symptoms are believed to be an expression of the body's wisdom as it reacts to cure its own imbalance or disease. Other threads or concepts common to most forms of alternative medicine include the following:

- An internal self-healing process exists within each person.
- People are responsible for making their own decisions regarding their health care.
- Nature, time, and patience are the great healers.

Two Paradigms, Possibly Complementary

Western medicine has made astonishing advances in the past two centuries. The fundamental physical mechanisms of the body are known and, perhaps, understood. Childbirth, once the primary cause of death in women and children, has been rendered almost routine. The processes of infection and disease transmission have been discovered and controlled. Physicians routinely make astonishing repairs to broken bones, brains, and hearts. A remarkable success has been achieved in countering the acute problems of most peoples' health. But as these acute illnesses and injuries become less prevalent and life-threatening, more chronic problems are emerging: cancer, heart disease, diabetes, mental and spiritual illnesses. It is against these types of challenges that alternative medicine can be used most effectively.

When Einstein introduced his theory of relativity in 1905, our way of viewing the universe changed dramatically. Einstein said that all matter is energy, energy and matter are interchangeable, and all matter is connected at the subatomic level. No single entity could be affected without all connecting parts being affected. In this view, the universe is not a giant clock, but a living web. The human body is animated by an integrated energy called the *life force*. The life force sustains the physical body but is also a spiritual entity that is linked to a higher being or infinite source of energy. When the life force flows freely throughout the body, a person experiences optimal health and vitality. When the life force is blocked or weakened, organs, tissues, and cells are deprived of the energy they need to function at their full potential, and illness or disease results. As the costs of conventional medicine grow and people continue to suffer from chronic illnesses and degenerative diseases, alternative medicine is a more and more appropriate system for the maintenance of this life.

What Are the Theoretical Foundations of the Two Systems?

In understanding and comparing conventional and alternative medicine, it is helpful to study the assumptions that are basic to their theories, practices, and research. These include assumptions about the origin of disease, the meaning of health, the healing process, and the nature of healthy living (see Table 1.3).

TABLE 1.3   Paradigms of Medicine

	Conventional Medicine	Alternative Medicine
Mind/body/spirit are...	separate	one
The body is...	a machine	a living microcosm or universe
Disease results when...	parts break	energy/life force becomes unbalanced
The role of medicine is to...	combat disease	restore mind/body/ spirit harmony
Approach is to...	treat and suppress symptoms	search for patterns of disharmony or imbalance
Focuses on...	parts/matter	whole/energy
Treatments...	attempt to "fix" broken parts	support self-healing
Primary interventions include...	drugs, surgery	diet, exercise, herbs, stress management, social support
A system of...	sick care	health care

Origin of Disease

Biomedicine and alternative medicine have widely divergent beliefs about the origin of disease. Biomedicine was shaped by the observations that bacteria were responsible for producing disease and its damage and that antitoxins and vaccines could improve a person's ability to ward off the undesirable effects of these harmful agents. Armed with this knowledge, physicians began to conquer a large number of devastating infectious diseases. As the science developed, physicians came to believe that germs and genes caused disease and once the offending pathogen, metabolic error, or chemical imbalance was found, all diseases would eventually yield to the appropriate vaccine, antibiotic, or chemical compound.

Conventional medicine has also been influenced by Darwin's concept of survival of the fittest, which says that all life is a constant struggle and that only the most successful competitors survive. When this concept is applied to medicine it results in the belief that we live under constant attack by the thousands of microorganisms that, in the Western view, cause most diseases. People must defend themselves and counterattack with treatments that kill the enemy.

Based on this assumption, symptoms are regarded as harmful manifestations that should be suppressed. For example, a headache is an annoyance that should be eliminated, and a fever is an attack on the body that should be countered by the use of medications.

Alternative medicine is based on the belief that a life force or energy flows through and sustains each person. Balance and harmony should be fostered among organs in the body, among body systems, and with other individuals, society, and the environment. A balanced organism presents a strong native defense against external insults like bacteria, viruses, and trauma. When the life force or energy is blocked or weakened, the vitality of organs and tissues is reduced, oxygen is diminished, waste products accumulate, and organs and tissues degenerate. Symptoms are the body's way of communicating that the life force has been blocked or weakened and that a compromised immune system has resulted. Disease is not necessarily a surprise meeting with bacteria or a virus, since they surround us constantly; rather, it is the end result of a series of events that began with a disruption of the life force.

Based on this assumption, symptoms are not suppressed unless they endanger life—a headache from an aneurysm or a fever above 105°F. Instead, symptoms are cooperated with because they express the body's wisdom as it reacts to cure its own disease. A headache is regarded as a signal that the whole system needs realignment, and a fever may be the result of the breakdown of bacterial proteins or toxins. When symptoms are suppressed, they are not resolved but merely held off, gathering energy for renewed expression as soon as the outside, curative force is removed.

The Meaning of Health

A healer from the Chinese, Indian, or Native American traditions would give very different opinions about the meaning of health from those given by a Western physician. The Western view of health, in the past, was often described as the absence of disease or other abnormal conditions. That definition expanded to include the view that health is not a static condition; the body undergoes constant change and adaptation to both internal and external challenges. The majority of conventional medical practitioners would define health as a state of well-being. They may disagree, however, about who determines well-being—the health professional or the individual.

Those practicing alternative medicine describe health as a condition of wholeness, balance, and harmony of the body, mind, emotions, and spirit. Health is not a concrete goal to be achieved; rather, it is a lifelong process that represents growth toward potential, an inner feeling of aliveness. Physical aspects include the optimal functioning of all body systems. Emotional aspects include the ability to feel and express the entire range of human emotions. Mental aspects include feelings of self-worth, a positive identity, a sense of accomplishment, and the ability to appreciate and create. Spiritual health is experienced within the self, with others, and as a part of society. Self-related components are the development of moral values and finding a meaningful purpose in life. Spiritual factors relating to others include the search for meaning through relationships and the feeling of connectedness with others and with an external power often identified as God or the divine source. Societal aspects of spiritual health can be understood as a common humanity and a belief in the fundamental sacredness and unity of all life. These beliefs motivate people toward truth and a sense of fairness and justice to all members of society. The World Health Organization (WHO) states, "the existing definition of health should include the spiritual aspect and that health care should be in the hands of those who are fully aware of and sympathetic to the spiritual dimension."

The Healing Process

The curative process is another example of divergent viewpoints. Conventional medicine promotes the view that external treatments—drugs, surgery, radiation—cure people, and practitioners are trained to fix or repair broken parts. The focus is on the disease process or abnormal conditions.

Alternative practitioners look at conditions that block the life force and keep it from flowing freely through the body. Healing occurs when balance and harmony are restored. The focus is on the health potential of the person rather than the disease problem. The cure model and the healing model are presented with greater detail in Chapter 2, "How Does Alternative Medicine Work?"

The Nature of Healthy Living

Conventional and alternative medical systems have different perspectives on the promotion of health. Conventional medicine focuses on disease prevention. Consumers are taught how to decrease their risk of cancer, cardiac disorders, and other life-threatening diseases that cause most premature deaths in Western society. As important as these behaviors are, however, disease prevention is only one piece of health promotion.

Health promotion from the alternative perspective is a lifelong process that focuses on optimal development of our physical, emotional, mental, and spiritual selves. An individual's worldviews, values, lifestyles, and health beliefs are considered to be of critical importance. People are encouraged to adopt healthier lifestyles, to accept increased responsibility for their own well-being, and to learn how to handle common health problems on their own through greater self-reliance.

Research Comparing the Two Systems

Scientific beliefs rest not just on facts, but on paradigms—broad views of how these facts are related and organized. Differences of opinion between groups of researchers are at least partly a reflection of the different scientific paradigms each group uses. This understanding may provide some insight into the ongoing conflict between quantitative and qualitative researchers, nursing and medical researchers, Western and Eastern researchers, and conventional and alternative medical researchers. A common, yet seemingly almost invisible, presumption is that the "experts" of conventional medicine are entitled and qualified to pass judgment on the scientific and therapeutic merits of alternative therapies. However, since the paradigms of the systems are so different, they are truly not qualified. Just like the use of the therapies themselves, understanding alternative medicine from a research perspective requires the blending of multiple techniques and points of view.

Three Approaches to Research

Particulate-deterministic, or quantitative, research represents the principles of Western scientific method, which include formulating and testing hypotheses and then rejecting or accepting the hypotheses. Every question is reduced to the smallest possible part. Results can be replicated and generalized. Outcomes can be predicted and controlled. Particulate-deterministic research is said to be objective in that the observer is separate from those being observed. Another part of this objective paradigm is that all information can be derived from physically measurable data. This type of research has been extremely effective for isolating the factors that cause disease and for developing cures. On the other hand, it cannot explain the whole person as an integrated unit.

Interactive-integrative research studies the context and meaning of interactive variables as these variables form patterns that reflect the whole. Researchers observe, document, analyze, and qualify the interactive relationship of variables. In physics, it is believed that objectivity of measurement is ultimately not possible. The Heisenberg uncertainty principle states that the act of observing phenomena unavoidably influences the behavior of the phenomena being observed. The interactive-integrative paradigm embraces this unity of measurement and measured. Another part of the paradigm relates to the belief that interactions between living organisms and environments are transactional, multidirectional, and synergistic—they cannot be reduced. The holistic belief that the whole is greater than the sum of the parts is basic to the interactive-integrative paradigm.

The unitary-transformative approach to research represents a significant paradigm shift. A phenomenon is viewed as an integral, self-organizing unit embedded in a larger, self-organizing unit. Change is nonlinear and unpredictable, as systems move through organization and disorganization. Knowledge is a function of both the observer and observed and is primarily a matter of pattern recognition. Knowledge is personal in that it includes thoughts, values, feelings, choices, and purpose.

Just as conventional and alternative medicine complement one another, so do multiple perspectives of research. Some research explores patterns about how little is known (interactive-integrative), while other research validates new knowledge and predicts outcomes of interventions (particulate-deterministic). Yet other research may help us understand such aspects as the mutuality of patient/healer encounters (unitary-transformative). All paradigms are needed to further scientific knowledge.

The Limits of Western Thinking

Those who limit themselves to Western scientific research have virtually ignored anything that cannot be perceived by the five senses and repeatedly measured or quantified. Research is dismissed as superstitious and invalid if it cannot be scientifically explained by cause and effect. Many continue to cling with an almost religious fervor to this cultural paradigm about the power of science—more specifically, the power that science gives them. By dismissing non-Western scientific paradigms as inferior at best and inaccurate at worst, the most entrenched members of the conventional medical research community try to counter the threat that alternative therapies and research pose to their work, their well-being, their worldviews.

And yet, biomedical research cannot explain many of the phenomena that concern alternative practitioners regarding caring-healing processes. When therapies such as acupuncture or homeopathy are observed to result in a physiological or clinical response that cannot be explained by the biomedical model, many have tried to deny the results rather than modify the scientific model. In contrast to the biomedical perspective, Buckminster Fuller, an American architect and inventor, said, "Eighty percent of reality cannot be perceived or detected through the five senses." If researchers limit themselves to the five senses, they will never come to understand human energy fields, electromagnetic fields, thoughts as a form of energy, or the healing power of prayer.

Conventional medicine also believes that procedures and substances must pass a double-blind study to be proven effective. As a testing method, the double-blind study examines a single procedure or substance in isolated, controlled conditions, and measures its results against those of a procedure or substance known to be inactive. This approach is based on the presumption that single factors cause and reverse illness, and that these factors can be studied alone and out of context. Alternative medicine, however, believes that no single factor causes anything, nor can a magic substance single-handedly reverse illness. Multiple factors contribute to illness, and multiple interventions work together to promote healing. The double-blind method is incapable of reconciling this degree of complexity and variation.

Although major alternative medical systems may not have a great deal of quantitative research, they are generally not experimental. They rely on well-developed clinical observational skills and experience that is guided by their explanatory models. Likewise, 70 to 85 percent of biomedical practices are guided by observation and experience and have not been tested quantitatively. While new medicines must have rigorous proof of efficacy and safety before clinical use, the use of tests, procedures, and treatments are not similarly constrained. A tiny fraction of new devices undergoes formal review by the Food and Drug Administration before marketing approval. Western physicians, like alternative practitioners, use the same well-developed clinical observational skills and experience, guided by their explanatory biomedical model. Thus, the argument really becomes one of cultural bias rather than scientific method.

Meticulous documentation for all claims that are made by the various therapies is beyond the scope of this guide. The National Center for Complementary and Alternative Medicine at the National Institutes of Health (nccam.nih.gov) has been mandated to facilitate the evaluation of alternative medical treatments, most typically conducted at universities and medical schools, and to provide the public with this information. There may be a wait for new knowledge from quantum physics and psychoneuroimmunology before alternative medicine can be understood in terms of the biomedical model. Successful alternative therapies, however, should not be withheld from the public while research is debated.

THE ABSOLUTE MINIMUM

■ Western healthcare consumers, finding traditional therapies ineffective, unfriendly, and overly concerned with symptoms and not causes, have turned to alternative therapies in ever-increasing numbers—almost 50% of Americans in recent years.

■ Most alternative therapies focus on releasing the healing powers within the body, rather than creating healing through the application of outside forces like surgery, technology, or pharmaceuticals.

■ Although the profoundly different natures of the two systems make comparison research hard to come by, the research done in the past 10–15 years provides compelling evidence that alternative therapies create healing, even if the way they do so is not always clear.

RESOURCES: INSTITUTION-AFFILIATED CENTERS OF RESEARCH ON ALTERNATIVE MEDICINE

Institution	Specialty of Center
Bastyr University, Bethel, WA	HIV/AIDS
Columbia University, New York, NY	Women's health issues
Harvard Medical School, Boston, MA	General medical conditions
Kessler Institute for Rehabilitation, West Orange, NJ	Stroke and neurological conditions
Palmer Center for Chiropractic Research, Davenport, IA	Chiropractic
Stanford University Palo Alto, CA	Aging
University of Arizona Health Science Center Tucson	Pediatric conditions
University of California Davis	Asthma, allergy, and immunology
University of Maryland School of Medicine Baltimore	Pain
University of Michigan Ann Arbor	Cardiovascular diseases
University of Texas Health Science Center	Houston Cancer
University of Virginia Charlottesville	Pain

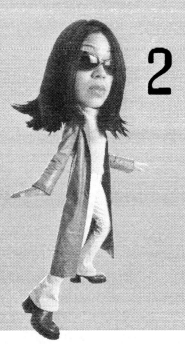

2

HOW DOES ALTERNATIVE MEDICINE WORK?

At the core of all of the alternative therapies discussed in this guide are four concepts: balance, spirituality, energy, and breath. In one way or another, each of the methods discussed in the remaining chapters of this book relies on those central principles, which we'll explore in this chapter before getting to our detailed examination of each of the therapies.

Balance

An expression in the Native American culture, "walking in balance," describes the philosophy of a peaceful coexistence and harmony with all aspects of life. This concept of balance is found in all cultures throughout time. For optimal wellness, the mental, physical, emotional, and spiritual components of health need to be balanced, and equilibrium is needed among all the components. Walking in balance is a learned skill and one that must be practiced regularly to engage in the process of healthful living. This concept of balance appears again and again throughout the various alternative healing practices.

Circadian Rhythms

Universal rhythmic cycles are observed in plants, animals, and people and are referred to as *circadian rhythms*. The word circadian derives from the Latin, *circa diem,* which means "about a day." Circadian rhythms are regular fluctuations of activity and rest in a variety of physiologic processes that occur every 23–27 hours. Most familiar are the 24-hour temperature and sleep patterns. Less well known is the fact that immunity to viruses and infection is lower in the early hours of the morning, when most people are usually sleeping. Blood also clots more slowly in to late day than in the early hours of the morning. Taking these factors into consideration, hospitals might do well to schedule elective surgeries later in the day rather than the typical early morning schedule.

The constant rhythmic processes bring about a dynamic, healthy balance in our bodies. The beating and relaxation of the heart help the cardiovascular system regulate blood pressure throughout the body. The inspiration and expiration of breath in the respiratory system allow for gas exchange. The nervous system has a number of rhythmic processes including nerve depolarization and repolarization, systemic excitation and recovery, and sleep and waking cycles. Attention to the rhythmic nature of one's own being reveals an intimate relationship with the rhythms of the surrounding natural world.

Musical Rhythms

Health is about balance or harmony of body, mind, and spirit. In a state of optimal health, all frequencies are in harmony, like a finely tuned piano. In fact, music is often used in healing, from the ancient sounds of the drum, rattle, bone flute, and other primitive instruments to the current use of music as a prescription for health. The Chinese are producing musical recordings with some curious titles. *Obesity, Constipation,* and *Liver, Heart, and Lungs* are three examples. Most of the recordings use traditional Chinese instruments and are to be listened to or "taken" as an individual would take an herbal medicine, to help cope with problems or strengthen the organs described in the titles. For headaches and migraines, the Japanese suggest Mendelssohn's *Spring Song*, Dvorak's *Humoresque*, or even a dose of George Gershwin's *An American in Paris*. At hospitals throughout India, traditional Indian music is used medicinally to balance the rhythms of the body. Western researchers have lately established the healing and creative powers of sound and music in general and in particular Mozart's music, which seems to have a special ability to improve learning and healing. It is thought that his music facilitates certain complex neuronal patterns in the cerebral cortex, increasing left-brain activities such as logical thinking, as well as strengthening the creative right-brain processes. Vibrating sounds create energy fields of resonance and movement in the surrounding space. These energies are absorbed and subtly alter one's internal rhythms.

HEALTHFUL MUSIC

- In a study on the effects of music on nearly 97,000 people before, during, and after surgery, 97 percent reported that listening to slow baroque or classical music helped them relax and reduced their postoperative disorientation.

- Twenty-seven people with rheumatoid arthritis used Guided Imagery and Music (GIM) for 18 weeks and reported a reduction in both pain and psychological distress as well as improvement in walking.

- Children with attention deficit disorder (ADD) who listened to Mozart were able to improve their attention, have better control over their moods, lessen their impulsivity, and improve their social skills.

- At the Ireland Cancer Center at the University Hospital of Cleveland, 19 children demonstrated a significant increase in salivary immunoglobulin A (IgA) after a single half-hour music therapy session. IgA, an antibody in saliva, is a principle marker in enhanced resistance to disease.

- In a study of 20 developmentally disabled children, most of whom had cerebral palsy, 75% demonstrated improved attention, reduced hypersensitivity, and improved coordination after listening to baroque compositions by Vivaldi and Bach.

Spirituality

Spiritual healing techniques and spiritually based health care systems are among the most ancient healing practices. Spirit is the liveliness, richness, and beauty of one's life. Spirituality is the drive to become everything one can be, and it is bound to intuition, creativity, and motivation. It is the dimension that involves relationships with oneself, with others, and with a higher power. It involves finding significant meaning in the entirety of life, including illness and death.

The materialism of North American culture of the 1980s has given way to a period of reflectiveness. People are searching for a "wholeness" in their lives and a way to allow their innermost selves to grow and expand. Spiritual healing practices guide people to places within themselves they did not know existed, through techniques as ancient as prayer, contemplation, meditation, drumming, storytelling, and mythology. In consciously awakening the energies of the spirit, people are able to move toward healing places and sacred moments in their lives.

Spirituality and Suffering

During periods of stress, illness, or crisis, people search for meaning and purpose in their pain and suffering. They ask questions like "Why am I sick?" or "Why did this bad thing happen to me?" This spiritual quest for meaning can lead to insight and healing or to fear and isolation. In the words of Buddhist philosopher Ken Wilber,

> A person who is beginning to sense the suffering of life, is, at the same time, beginning to awaken to deeper realities, truer realities. For suffering smashes to pieces the complacency of our normal fictions about reality, and forces us to become alive in a special sense—to see carefully, to feel deeply, to touch ourselves and our world in ways we have heretofore avoided. It has been said, and truly I think, that suffering is the first grace.

Spirituality is not religion. Spirituality, however, is the search for wholeness and purpose that underlies the world's religions. Remove the dogma, the politics, and the cultural influence from any of the world's religions, and you find the same questions, the same seeking, and the same answers. The concept of spirituality does not undermine any religion but rather enhances all religions by illuminating their commonalities and the commonality among all people. It makes us far more similar to each other than it makes us different.

Spiritual Guides

Many traditions also speak of spiritual guides. Some of us think of them as guardian angels, others as Beings of Light who guide people through near-death experiences.

Although no Western scientific evidence supports the existence of angels, one can find phenomenological evidence. Many first-person accounts of near-death occurrences involve angels and similar experiences from people of different ages, from diverse cultures, with different personal and religious beliefs.

note

A number of books provide more information about angels including *Angels, an Endangered Species* by Malcolm Godwin, *A Book of Angels* by Sophy Burnham, and *Many Lives, Many Masters* by Brian Weiss.

Energy

The concept of energy has been recognized for centuries, and in most cultures. Many ancient and current cultures have great respect for the subtle and unseen forces in life. Most spiritual traditions share the belief that energy is the bridge between spirit and physical being. Meditation and prayer are believed to be subtle energy phenomena that represent contact with the spiritual dimension.

Chinese Taoist scholars believed that energy, not matter, was the basic building material of the universe. Albert Einstein and other physicists proved that matter and energy are the same and that energy is not only the raw material of the cosmos but also the glue that holds it together. Modern scientists now look at the universe in terms of forces instead of tiny particles of matter. Their experimental findings are similar to the intuitive observations of China's ancient scholars. Everything in the world—animate and inanimate—is made of energy. People are beings of energy, living in a universe composed of energy.

Although Western scientists agree that energy comprises all things, when this notion is applied to the human body they do not yet fully agree that a distinct energy system exists within the physical body. In order for energy to be "real," it must be measurable by scientific instruments. By this logic, of course, brain waves did not exist prior to the invention of EEG equipment! Since technology is not yet capable of measuring all the energy fields in the body, references to energy are conspicuously absent in conventional medicine. Some researchers believe that in the not-too-distant future, Western scientists will begin to agree that humans are a matrix of interacting multidimensional energy fields.

Life Force

For more than 2,000 years, various practitioners around the world have insisted that a person is more than the physical body. According to these healers, a "life force" of subtle energy surrounds and permeates every person. Energy is viewed as the force that integrates the body, mind, and spirit; it is that which connects everything. The Chinese call this life force *qi* (also spelled *chi*), the Ancient Greeks called it *pneuma*, and the Hindus give it the name *prana*. Whatever the culture, it is believed that the life force is both self-nurturing and self-sustaining. In other words, physical activities such as eating, work, and rest, as well as nonphysical aspects of life such as will, motivation, feelings, desires, and a sense of purpose in life, are both made possible by qi and responsible for creating more qi. Most schools of thought basically agree on the following points regarding energy:

- Energy comes from one universal source.
- Movement of energy is the basis of all life.
- Matter is an expression of energy, and vice versa.
- All things are manifestations of energy.
- The entire earth has energetic and metabolic qualities.
- People are composed of multiple, interacting energy fields that extend out into the environment.
- People's relationships with one another are shaped by the interactions of their energies.

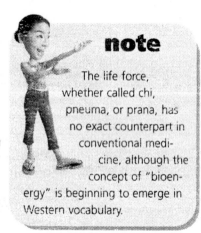

note

The life force, whether called chi, pneuma, or prana, has no exact counterpart in conventional medicine, although the concept of "bioenergy" is beginning to emerge in Western vocabulary.

Chakras

The Hindu concept of *chakras* (a Sanskrit word for "spinning wheel") describes seven major energy centers within the physical body. Chakras have been described by most eastern cultures and several South American cultures (such as the Mayan culture) for thousands of years. Chakras are major centers of both electromagnetic activity and circulation of vital energy. They are usually thought of as funnels of perpetually rotating energy and are considered the gateways through which energy enters and leaves the body. Each chakra in the body is recognized as a focal point of life force relating to physical, emotional, mental, and spiritual aspects of people and they are the network through which the body, mind, and spirit interact as one holistic system. Figure 2.1 illustrates the sites of the chakras in the body.

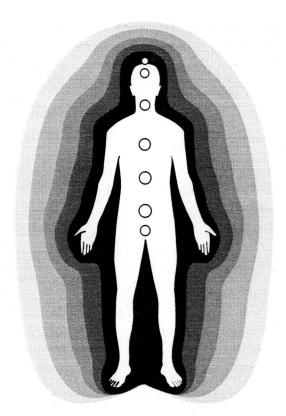

The concept of chakras may be foreign to the Western scientific mind, but they are not completely unknown to those familiar with Judeo-Christian artwork. For centuries, the crown chakra, which signifies a conscious awareness of the divine, has been painted as a halo over those who are consciously aware of a divine presence in their lives.

The seven main chakras are vertically aligned up the center of the body from the base of the pelvis to the top of the head. Each chakra has its own individual characteristics and functions and each has a corresponding relationship to various organs and structures of the body, to one of the endocrine glands, as well as to one of the seven colors of the rainbow spectrum. The characteristics of the seven major chakras are described in Table 2.1. Of the many smaller chakras throughout the body, the most significant are in the palms of the hands. The hand chakras are considered extensions of the heart chakra and, as such, radiate healing and soothing energies. Spiritual healers who practice the laying on of hands concentrate energy in their hand chakras. All the chakras have purpose, function, and frequency as described here:

■ Chakras regulate the human energy system, as well as maintain the equilibrium of health (purpose).

■ Linking body, mind, and spirit and the exchange of energy (function).

■ The operation of each chakra at its own optimum frequency; generally the lower the chakra on the body, the lower its frequency; if one is out of sync, all others will be too (frequency) .

Table 2.1 The Seven Major Chakras

1. Root Chakra

Location	Base of the spine
Center of	Physical vitality, urge to survive
Gland	Adrenal glands
Organs/structures	Kidneys, bladder, spine
Color	Red

2. Sexual or Navel Chakra

Location	Slightly below the navel, in front of the sacrum
Center of	Sexual energy, ego, extrasensory perception
Gland	Gonads
Organs/structures	Reproductive organs, legs
Color	Orange

3. Solar Plexus Chakra

Location	Slightly above the navel
Center of	Unrefined emotions, urge for power
Gland	Pancreas
Organs/structures	Stomach, liver, gall-bladder
Color	Yellow

4. Heart Chakra

Location	Middle of the chest, at the height of the heart
Center of	Unconditional affection, compassion, devotion, love, spiritual growth
Gland	Thymus
Organs/structures	Heart, liver, lungs, circulatory system
Color	Emerald

5. Throat Chakra

Location	Throat area
Center of	Communication, self-expression, creativity
Gland	Thyroid
Organs/structures	Throat, upper lungs, digestive tract,
Color	Blue

6. Third Eye Chakra

Location	Middle of the forehead, a little higher than the eyebrows
Center of	The will, intellect, spirit, spiritual awakening, visualization
Gland	Pituitary
Organs/structures	Spine, lower brain, left eye, nose
Color	Purple

7. Crown Chakra

Location	At the top of the head at the fontenal
Center of	Highest level of consciousness or enlightenment, intuition, direct spiritual vision
Gland	Pineal
Organs/structures	Upper brain, right eye
Color	Golden-white

The main purpose in working with and understanding the chakras is to create integration and wholeness within people. The chakras are the "doorways" through which energy is distributed to cells, tissues, and organs. If chakras stop functioning properly, the intake of energy will be disturbed and the body organs served by that chakra will not get their needed supply of energy. Eventually organ functioning will be disrupted, leading to weakened organs with a diminished immune defense. If this process continues, the end result will be dysfunction and disease. Dr. Dean Ornish, well-known for his program to reverse blocked coronary arteries through diet, exercise, support groups, and meditation—without surgery or drugs—believes that a closed heart chakra (unresolved anger and fear) is related to the closed coronary arteries. Consequently, the meditation technique he incorporates into his program involves opening the heart chakra. His holistic approach has now become a recognized program practiced nationwide.

Aura

Closely related to the chakras is the concept of aura. The aura is the energy field surrounding each person as far as the outstretched arms and from head to toe. This energy field is both an information center and a highly sensitive perceptual system that transmits and receives messages from the internal and external environment. Each of the seven layers of the auric field is associated with a chakra; the first layer is related to the first chakra, and so on. Each layer has physical, mental, emotional, and spiritual dimensions and purposes, and the layers function together through the transmission of energy. (Refer back to Figure 2.1 and see Table 2.2 for the characteristics and structure of the auric field.) Virtually every alternative healing therapy has a way of interpreting the body's subtle energy.

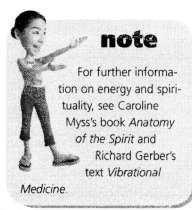

note

For further information on energy and spirituality, see Caroline Myss's book *Anatomy of the Spirit* and Richard Gerber's text *Vibrational Medicine*.

TABLE 2.2   Seven Layers of the Auric Field

Level 1. Etheric Body

Location	One-quarter inch to two inches beyond the physical body
Center of	Physical functioning and physical sensation
Color	Light blue to gray

Level 2. Emotional Body

Location	One to three inches beyond the physical body; roughly follows the outline of the physical body
Center of	Emotional aspects of person
Color	All colors of the rainbow

Level 3. Mental Body

Location	Three to eight inches beyond the physical body
Center of	Instinct, intellect, intuition
Color	Bright yellow with additional colors superimposed

Level 4. Astral Body

Location	Six to 16 inches beyond the physical body
Center of	Love
Color	Same colors as in level 3 but infused with the rose light of love

Level 5. Etheric Template Body

Location	Eighteen to 24 inches beyond the physical body
Center of	Higher will connected with divine will, speaking, listening, work, taking responsibility for our actions
Color	Clear lines on cobalt blue background

Level 6. Celestial Body

Location	Twenty-four to 33 inches beyond the physical body
Center of	Celestial love, spiritual ecstasy, protection and nurturance of all life
Color	Shimmering pastel colors

Level 7. Causal Body

Location	Thirty to 42 inches, forming an egg shape around body
Center of	Higher mind; integration of spiritual and physical body
Color	Shimmering gold threads

Meridians

A person's vital energy is not simply radiated outward; it also has patterns of circulation within the body, referred to as the *meridian system*. Meridians are a network of energy circuits or lines of force that run vertically through the body, connecting all parts. Meridians may be understood more clearly if they are compared to a major city's highway system, with entrance and exit ramps, merging roads, and connecting surface streets. If a flood blocks an exit ramp, the streets served by this ramp are inaccessible, affecting the people who live and work on those streets. What's more, the traffic may be backed up on the highway waiting for the ramp to reopen, affecting the people stuck in that traffic jam. Meridians operate this way in a person's body. If some kind of blockage affects your hip, for example, the pathways of energy leading to that hip get "backed up." Pain or discomfort restricts the motion of the hip, which puts a different strain on the foot, and the foot in a different position creates a strain on other sets of muscles. Changes in the body's general posture affect the positions of the internal organs, restricting nutrition to the organs, altering organ function, and thereby changing the body's balance. As the body and mind are affected, the person will think and feel differently, leading to more tension and more changes.

Each meridian passes close to the skin's surface at places called *hsueh*, which means cave or hollow and is translated as point or acupuncture point. Since each meridian is associated with an internal organ, the acupuncture points offer surface access to the internal organ systems. The flow of qi can be strengthened or weakened by manipulating specific points. Keeping the flow of energy open contributes to a state of balance and health.

The California Institute for Human Science is the American center for research on a machine called the AMI, an acronym for "apparatus for meridian identification." The AMI measures the flow of ions through the body and in 10 minutes can give a complete evaluation of the condition of a person's meridian system and the corresponding internal organs related to those meridians. This stream of ions is not vital energy or qi itself. Rather, it is a secondary electromagnetic effect of qi—in a sense, its imprint in the physical domain. The AMI is now becoming available for wide distribution as a diagnostic tool in medicine.

Energy Concentration

The mind's energy, or willpower, can be developed to control the body's energy system to an extraordinary degree. Healers can concentrate and manipulate energy in remarkable ways. Doctors at the Menninger Clinic compared average people to healers by measuring the electrical field on their hands. Ordinary people varied from 0 to 50 millivolts of energy in their hands. (A millivolt is 1/1,000 of a volt.) When he measured the electrical energy of the hands of people who worked as traditional healers, he found that they all produced at least 4 volts of energy, more than 80 times more energy than the average person. One Chinese *qi gong* master produced 200 volts, the equivalent of 4,000 times more energy. The investigators also attempted to trace the source of the healers' electricity. It seemed to come from the central body in the area between the solar plexus and the lower abdomen. The Chinese refer to this spot as the *tan dien* or the home of qi, and the Hindu refer to it as the solar plexus chakra or the seat of prana.

Grounding and Centering

Two terms common in various healing practices and related to energy and balance are grounding and centering. *Grounding*, as its name suggests, relates to one's connection with the ground and, in a broader sense, to one's whole contact with reality. Being grounded suggests stability, security, independence, having a solid foundation, and living in the present rather than escaping into dreams. It means having a mature sense of responsibility. Much of the sense of grounding comes from identification with the lower half of the body—the parts of being that are less conscious and have more instinctive functions of movement. Learning to breathe into the belly, for example, is vital for grounding, for if the breath is shallow, contact with feelings and reality is limited. Many of the practices in this text, such as biofield therapies, mind-body techniques, and spiritual therapies, help to increase your groundedness.

Centering refers to the process of bringing oneself to the center or middle. When people are centered, they are fully connected to the part of their bodies where all energies meet. Centering is the process of focusing the mind on the center of energy, usually in the navel or solar plexus chakra. All movement in the body originates from this center, providing the meeting point for body and mind. It is commonly considered the "earth" center, for it gathers energy from the earth rising up through the legs. Centering can be achieved through movement, as in T'ai Chi, or it can be found in stillness, as in meditation. Being centered allows one to operate intuitively, with awareness, and to channel energy throughout the body.

Breath

Breath is at the center of all spiritual and religious traditions. In many languages the words for spirit and breath are one and the same—Sanskrit *prana*, Hebrew *ruach*, Greek *pneuma*, and Latin *spiritus*. In Christianity, the Holy Spirit is referred to as "the breath of life." To in-spire, or take in spirit, not only means to inhale but also to encourage, motivate, and give hope. To ex-pire, or lose spirit, not only means to exhale but also to die, cease to exist, to end or be destroyed.

In Eastern cultures, when air is inhaled, so is vital energy, which flows into the body to nourish and enliven. In Traditional Chinese Medicine, the exhalation is considered the yin part of the breath, and the inhalation is yang. It is impossible to only breathe in without breathing out or to breathe out without breathing in. It is the continuous dynamic balance of yin and yang that contributes to health and well-being. Most of the healing traditions worldwide believe breath is the most important function of life, and breathing restrictions lead to dysfunction and disease.

THE BREATH OF LIFE, AND GOOD HEALTH

In Western culture, the breath has been considered simply a mechanical, metabolic function of the body. Scientists are now beginning to recognize that breath can be used for healing, improving the body's self-repair processes, and reducing vulnerability to illness. Oxygen is toxic to viruses, bacteria, yeasts, and parasites in the body. Cancer cells find it more difficult to survive in an oxygen-rich environment. A 13-year study of longevity found that respiratory capacity was actually more significant than tobacco use, insulin metabolism, or cholesterol levels in determining the length of people's lives. People with cancer and other illnesses involved in breath therapy groups demonstrate an average 46% increase in the levels of immunoglobulin A (IgA) immediately after the breathing sessions. IgA is the body's first line of defense against germs entering through the mouth and nose that produce respiratory tract infections. It is, of course, only one component of the immune system, but the results demonstrate that breathing techniques can enhance immunity. Andrew Weil believes that "breath is the master key to health and wellness, a function we can learn to regulate and develop in order to improve our physical, mental, and spiritual well-being."

The breath is constantly adapting to accommodate the needs of the situation at hand. When people eat heavy meals or exercise rapidly, when their noses are congested or dry, or when their environment is filled with pleasant or unpleasant smells, breathing changes. Every change in posture has an effect on the combination of muscles used to breathe. Breath does not feel the same standing or sitting as when one is lying down. Breathing also changes under stress. For example, anxious people take shallow "chest" breaths, using only their chest muscles to inhale rather than their diaphragms. As a result, only the top part of their lungs fills with air, depriving the body of the optimal amount of oxygen.

Many people, even when feeling relaxed, breathe shallowly, which keeps them in a constant state of underoxygenation, which contributes to a decreased level of energy and increased vulnerability to illness. The typical shallow chest breath moves about half a pint of air, while a full abdominal breath can move eight to 10 times that amount. Forming healthy breathing habits can produce dramatic results. Probably no other single step that people can take will so profoundly and positively affect body, mind, and spirit. Deep breathing can counter stress. Just three deep, full belly breaths can move individuals from panic to calmness by increasing their oxygen intake. Much of perceived stress is worrying about the future or the past, and deep breathing is a great way to return people to the present. Twenty minutes of deep breathing exercises a day can lower blood pressure by increasing oxygen intake, which decreases the workload on your cardiovascular system.

TRY IT YOURSELF... FOCUSED BREATHING

BREATHING CLOUDS

Gently close your eyes and focus all your attention on the flow of air as you breathe in and exhale. After three to five breaths, visualize the air that you breathe into your lungs as a cloud of clean, pure, energized air. Tell yourself that the clean, fresh air that you breathe in through your nose has the power to clear your mind of distracting thoughts, as well as to cleanse and heal your body. As you slowly inhale this clean, pure air, feel the air enter your nose and travel up through the sinus cavity toward the top of your head. Visualize the air traveling down your spinal column and circulating throughout your abdominal area.

Now, as you exhale slowly and deeply, visualize that the air leaving your body is a dark, dirty cloud. This dark cloud of exhaled air symbolizes all your stressors, frustrations, and toxins. With each breath you take, allow the clean fresh air to enter and circulate and rejuvenate your body, while the exhalation of dark cloudy air helps to rid your body of its stress and tension. Repeat this breathing cycle for 5 to 10 minutes. As you continue this cycle of breathing clouds, visualize that as the body becomes more relaxed through the release of stress and tension, the color of the breath exhaled begins to change from dark to gray, perhaps even off-white, a message from your mind that it is cleansed and refreshed.

BREATHING ENERGY

From a point beneath your feet, bring energy up through the chakras to a place above your head. Then spiral it around you and down back to where you started. You can fill the spiral with light or color, whatever feels best for you. If you encounter someone around whom you tend to become drained, run the energy quickly up and down.

The Absolute Minimum

- Alternative therapies seek to access the native energy field of the body through breathing, physical manipulation, and conscious effort, and to harness that energy to create healing and increased health.

- Balance, spirituality, energy, and breath control lie at the center of most societies' healing traditions, and of all the alternative therapies described in this guide.

- Breathing exercises are the most accessible and inexpensive of all alternative treatments.

PART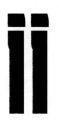

Non-Western Healing Methods

3

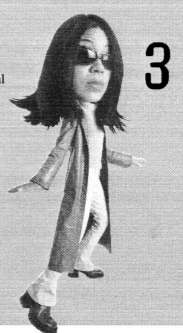

TRADITIONAL CHINESE MEDICINE

Chinese healers began the development of Traditional Chinese Medicine (TCM) more than 3,000 years ago. As a comprehensive health system, it has a range of applications from preventive health care and maintenance to diagnosis and treatment of acute and chronic disorders. Its treatments and diagnostic methods focus on balancing internal and external energies through diet, herbal treatments, acupuncture, and breathing techniques. Chinese healing practices have also spread, with variations, throughout other Asian countries, particularly Japan, Korea, Tibet, and Vietnam. In a few millennium of practice, TCM practitioners have evolved a system both subtle and dramatically effective, and one that, in China, is given as much if not more respect than Western medicine.

What Is Traditional Chinese Medicine?

Shen Nong the Fire Emperor, said to have lived from 2698 to 2598 BC, is considered the founder of herbal medicine in China. The written history of Traditional Chinese Medicine is more than 2,500 years old, starting with the text on internal medicine from Huang Di, the Yellow Emperor. Written long before the birth of Hippocrates, the father of Western medicine, the *Huang Di Nei Jing* (Yellow Emperor's Inner Classic) covers such principles as yin and yang, the five phases, the effects of the season, and treatments such as acupuncture and moxibustion (the burning of mugwort over inflamed and affected areas of the body).

TCM is associated with early Taoists and Buddhists who observed energy within themselves, in plants and animals, and throughout the cosmos. Based on a belief in the natural order of the universe and the direct correlation between the human body and the cosmos, this philosophy stresses the constant search for harmony and balance in an environment of constant change. By the close of the Han era (220 AD), the Chinese had a clear grasp of the nature of disease, preventive medicine, first aid, and dietetics, and had devised breathing practices to promote longevity.

During the fourth and fifth centuries AD, China's influence spread throughout Asia, and both Taoism and Buddhism had a marked impact on ideas about health. Sun Si Mian (581–682 AD), a famous physician, established himself as China's first medical ethicist. He advocated the need for rigorous scholarship, compassion toward patients, and high moral standards in physicians. In the eleventh century, TCM began to focus more on social phenomena, especially human relations and ethical behavior. Initially this orientation resulted in increased scientific medical study and publications.

As TCM developed further, however, people began to take for granted that a breakthrough in one realm of knowledge would eventually solve all problems of human existence. (As in the West, some assume that advances in technology will solve all problems.) Eventually, sociological methods were applied to medical problems, and clinical and empirical research reached a low point. Fortunately, the core of the scientific system was never obliterated, and this century has seen a worldwide revival of Traditional Chinese Medicine.

In China today, TCM is practiced in hospitals alongside Western medicine. Physicians not only study principles of anatomy, histology, biochemistry, bacteriology, and surgery but also acupuncture, acupressure, and herbal medicine. Patients can choose TCM or Western approaches alone or in combination to treat their particular problem.

TCM's development over thousands of years has yielded multiple philosophies, convergent concepts, and varied practices and treatments. It's impossible to separate the individual concepts and specific treatment approaches from the philosophy of the entire system. Prevention, diagnosis, and treatment of diseases are based on the concepts of *chi*, *yin* and *yang*, the five phases, the five seasons, and the three treasures. Often only isolated fragments of TCM emerge in the West, which may prevent more complete understanding and acceptance there.

Chi: The Energy in You and Me

The concept most central to TCM is *chi* (pronounced chee, and also spelled *qi*), which is translated as energy. Chi represents an invisible flow of energy that circulates through plants, animals, and people as well as the earth and sky. It is what maintains physiologic functions and the health and well-being of the individual. In TCM theory, energy is distributed throughout the body along a network of energy circuits or meridians, connecting all parts of the body. Obstructed chi flow in the human body can cause problems ranging from social difficulties to illness. Its effects are very individual—a person gets sick, has problems at work, or fights with family—and depend on each individual's unique chi. Certain TCM treatments such as meditation, exercise, and acupuncture are ways of enhancing or correcting the flow of chi.

Yin and Yang: Two Parts of the Whole

In the Taoist philosophy, wholeness is composed of the union of opposites—dark and light, soft and hard, female and male, slow and fast, and so forth. These opposite but complementary aspects are called *yin* and *yang*. Originally the terms designated geographical aspects such as the shady and sunny side of a mountain or the southern and northern bank of a river. In modern terms, they are used to characterize the polar opposites that exist in everything and make up the physical world. The traditional representation of the union of yin and yang is shown in Figure 3.1

FIGURE 3.1
Yin and yang: inseparable parts of the whole, each containing part of the other.

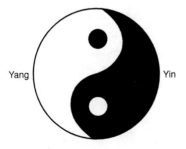

Yang   Yin

From the health perspective, the basis of well-being is the appropriate balance of yin and yang as they interact in the body. The imbalance of yin and yang is considered to be the cause of illness.

Yin is the general category for passivity and is like water, with a tendency to be cold and heavy. Yin uses fluids to moisten and cool our bodies. It provides for restfulness, as the body slows down and sleeps. Yin is associated more with substance than with energy. Things that are close to the ground are yin or more earthy. Yin is associated with the symptoms of coldness, paleness, low blood pressure, and chronic conditions. People with excess yin tend to catch colds easily, and are sedentary and sleepy.

Yang is the general category for activity and aggressiveness. It is like fire with its heating and circulating characteristics. Associated with things higher up or more heavenly, yang is the energy that directs movement and supports its substance. Symptoms such as redness in the face, fever, high blood pressure, and acute conditions are associated with yang. People with excess yang tend to be nervous and agitated and cannot tolerate much heat.

It must be understood that yin and yang cannot exist independently of each other. Nothing is either all yin or all yang. They are complementary and depend on each other for their very existence—without night there can be no day, without moisture there can be no dryness, and without cold there can be no heat. It is the interaction of yin and yang that creates the changes that keep the world in motion; summer leads to winter, night becomes day. Yin and yang are used in both the diagnosis and treatment of illness. For example, if a person is experiencing too much stress, usually understood as an excess of yang, more yin activities, such as meditation and relaxation, are the appropriate treatment.

The Five Phases: An Internal Cycle in Balance

As they studied the world around them, the Chinese perceived connections between major forces in nature and particular internal organ systems. Seeing similarities between natural elements and the body, early practitioners developed a concept of health care that encompassed both natural elements and body organs. This theory is known as the Five Phases Theory (*wu-hsing*). Five elements—fire, earth, metal, water, and wood—represent movement or energies that succeed one another in a dynamic relationship and in a continuous cycle of birth, life, and death. These elements do not represent static objects, since even mountains and rivers change constantly with time. In the Five Phases Theory, it is not the substances themselves that are important, but rather how they work together to make up the essential life force or chi.

The rhythm of events resembles a circle known as the Creation Cycle. In this cycle, wood burns to feed fire; fire's ashes produce earth; earth gives up its ore to create metal; metal causes condensation to bring forth water; and water nourishes and creates plants and trees, creating wood. Each element is related to a specific bodily system, as well as to a pair of internal organs—you guessed it, a yin organ and a yang organ. The yin organ is solid and dense, like the liver, while its yang partner is hollow or forms a pocket, like the gallbladder. Remember, no one element is the beginning or end—they flow together in an endless loop. It is the proper interaction of the organ partners that influences how well the entire body functions. The elements and their related systems and organs are shown in Table 3.1.

Table 3.1 Elements, Systems, and Organs of the Five Phases

Element	System	Yin Organ	Yang Organ
Wood	Toxin processing	Liver	Gallbladder
Fire	Circulation of blood, hormones, and food	Heart	Small Intestine
Earth	Digestion	Spleen & Pancreas	Stomach
Metal	Respiration and Elimination	Lungs	Large Intestine
Water	Elimination	Kidneys	Bladder

The Five Seasons: Balanced on the Outside

Just as the internal world of systems and organs is linked to the Five Phases, so too is the external world, specifically, the seasons and points of the compass. "But wait a minute," you say. "There are only four of each of those!" Remember, though, that the Chinese name for China means "The Middle Kingdom," and the fifth direction, the center, becomes obvious. Just as the center of the compass has a distinct identity in TCM, so does the center of the year—the late summer, when the agricultural cycle is at its peak, and after which most living things begin to decline into their Winter states.

The Chinese compass differs from the Western compass in one other way: Chinese culture places so much importance on the direction south that it, rather than north, is placed at the top of maps and compass roses. Just as south rules the top of the compass, it also represents summer, the "high noon" of the year and is linked to fire. West, the direction of the setting sun, is associated with autumn and metal, which is used to make tools for harvesting. North is linked to winter and water, the opposite of the element of fire and is seen as a period of dormancy. East, the direction of the rising sun, is associated with spring and with wood, which represents all growing things. The fifth and central element, earth, is related to the late summer season and a time of maturity. These relationships are shown in Figure 3.2.

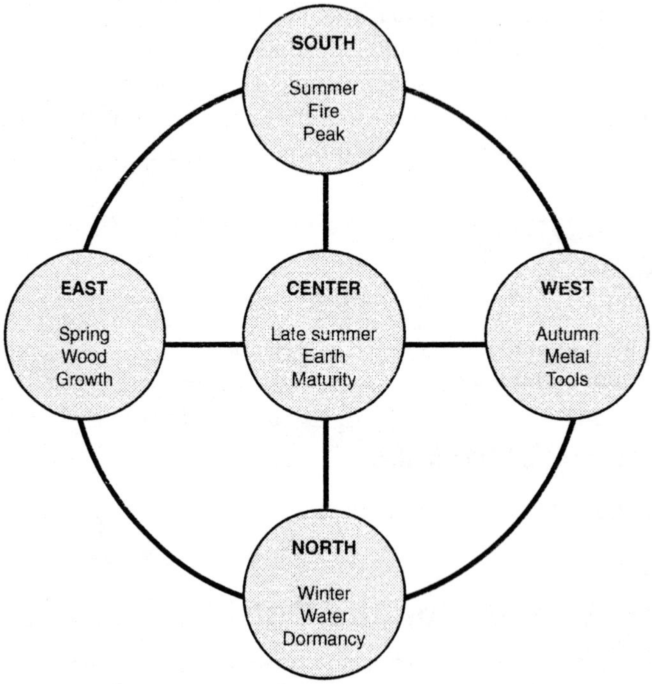

FIGURE 3.2

The Chinese compass rose gives not only direction, but also seasons, elements, and phases of the year.

SOUTH
Summer
Fire
Peak

EAST
Spring
Wood
Growth

CENTER
Late summer
Earth
Maturity

WEST
Autumn
Metal
Tools

NORTH
Winter
Water
Dormancy

Traditional Chinese Medicine traces the causes of disease to imbalances in these sets of five—elements, organs, seasons, and directions. If one component is overbearing and excessive, the system is thrown out of balance, and another component becomes weak and debilitated. It is a complex system of checks and balances that is often not easily grasped by those with a Western perspective. Diagnosis and treatment of illness depends on understanding the five elements, seasons, and directions and how they interact.

The Three Vital Treasures: Building Blocks of Life

The Chinese believe that a combination of life force elements make up the substance and functions of the body, mind, and spirit, which are fundamentally all one and the same. One way to understand this connection is to think of water with its wet, fluid nature. Compare that to ice, which not only appears different but feels hard and cold, and steam with its hot, gaseous nature. Despite the differences in appearance, the molecules are the same, they are simply in three different states. In the same way, body, mind, and spirit can be seen as different expressions of the same individual.

The Taoists call body, mind, and spirit the three "vital treasures." They are *jing*, meaning basic essence, *chi* meaning energy or life force, and *shen* meaning spirit and mind. The balance of their abundance or deficiency influences the state of health.

Jing is the essence with which people are born, similar to Western concepts of genes, DNA, and heredity. Essence is the gift of one's parents; it is the basic material in each cell that allows that cell to function. It is the bodily reserves that support life and must be restored by food and rest. Chi, as described previously, is the sustaining energy of all life. The vital treasure known as *shen* is the gift of heaven and represents spiritual and mental aspects of life. Shen comprises one's emotional well-being, thoughts, and beliefs. It is the radiance, or inner glow, that can be perceived by others. In order for people to be healthy, their physical, emotional, mental, and spiritual aspects must be balanced.

How Does Traditional Chinese Medicine Work?

The Chinese regard the body as a system that requires a balance of yin and yang energy to enjoy good health. Each part of the body is also thought of as an individual system that requires its own balance of yin and yang to function properly. TCM assumes that a balanced body has a natural ability to resist or cope with agents of disease. Symptoms are caused by an imbalance of yin and yang in some part of the body, and illness can develop if the imbalance persists for any length of time. Therefore, health is maintained by recognizing an imbalance before it becomes a disease. Chinese medicine holds that everything needed to restore health already exists in nature and that it is up to the individual, with or without the aid of a health practitioner, to free up energy and restore balance using diet, herbs, acupuncture, and other yin/yang treatments.

The Chinese believe that all living things—people, the earth, and the universe—are connected by cosmic energy. Thus the balance of chi in an individual is connected to the balance in the environment; the forces active within the world are the same forces active within the individual body. Simply put, nothing happens without consequence to something else. The concern for balance and harmony is not only reflected in the TCM approach to the individual but also in the view that the balance and well-being of the resources of the natural world and society are vital to the overall health of all who live on the earth. Practitioners never lose sight of the multifaceted relationship between individuals, communities, societies, and nature.

Traditional Chinese Diagnosis

The TCM practitioner has four diagnostic methods (*szu-chen*): inspection, auscultation/olfaction, inquiry, and palpation. These methods gather information about the five phases and their related body systems. The practitioner examines how the person eats, sleeps, thinks, works, relaxes, dreams, and imagines. No part of the self is considered a neutral bystander when the body is in a state of imbalance. All of this diagnostic information is compiled to arrive at a "pattern of disharmony," or *bian zheng*.

Inspection refers to the visual assessment of the spirit and physical body of patients. Spirit inspection or observation is an assessment of the person's overall appearance, especially the eyes, the complexion, and the quality of voice. Good spirit, even in the presence of serious illness, indicates a more positive prognosis.

Tongue diagnosis is a highly developed system of inspection of the physical body. The tongue is considered to be the visual gateway to the interior of the body. The whole body "lives" on the tongue, rather like a hologram. Different areas of the tongue correspond to the five phases and related organ systems as seen in Figure 3.3.

FIGURE 3.3

The microcosmic tongue— diagnostic information found in your mouth.

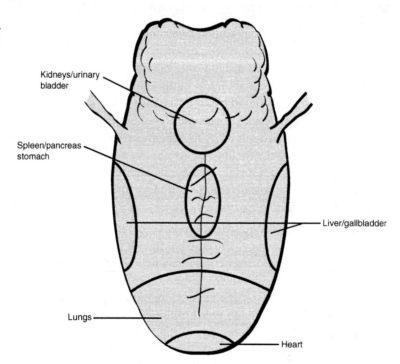

Kidneys/urinary bladder

Spleen/pancreas stomach

Liver/gallbladder

Lungs

Heart

The practitioner inspects the color, shape, markings, and coating of the tongue to gather information about the state of balance in the person's body. For example, a moist tongue with a thin white coating may signal the presence of a "cold" or yin illness whereas a dry, yellow or dark tongue may signal a "hot" or yang illness.

The second part of diagnosis consists of listening and smelling. Practitioners will listen to the quality of speech, breath, and other sounds their patients make, and they will observe other odors such as those from the breath and body, as well as excreta.

Types of sound are associated with the five phases and organ systems. How the person is breathing is a good indication of the status of the organs. Phases and organ systems are associated with specific odors such as sickly sweet, rotten, putrid, rancid, and scorched. Odors can arise from the skin itself or from the ears, nose, genitals, urine, stool, or bodily discharges. The breath may also have a distinctive odor. Usually the stronger the odor, the more serious the imbalance has become.

The third part of diagnosis, inquiry, is the process of taking a comprehensive health, social, emotional, and spiritual history. The practitioners question their patients not only about the complaint that brought them there, but also about many other factors, including sensations of hot and cold, perspiration, excreta, hearing, thirst, sleep, digestion, emotions, sexual drive, and energy level.

Palpation is the fourth diagnostic method and includes pulse examination and general touching and probing of the body, especially at the acupuncture points. Reading the pulses can provide key information about the person's condition. For example, a fast pulse might indicate a problem with an overactive heart or liver; a slow pulse might indicate a sluggish digestive system; pulses described as wide, flat, and soft may indicate a spleen problem; and narrow, forceful pulses might indicate a liver dysfunction. The locations of major points used in pulse diagnosis are illustrated in Figure 3.4. The pulse allows the practitioner to feel the quality of chi and blood at the different locations in the body.

FIGURE 3.4

Put your finger on it: major points used in pulse diagnosis.

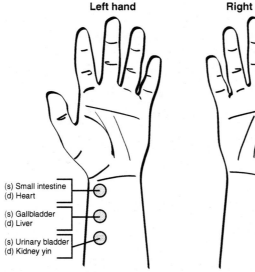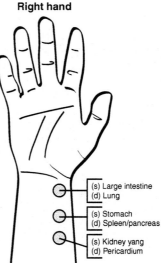

Left hand   **Right hand**

(s) Small intestine
(d) Heart

(s) Gallbladder
(d) Liver

(s) Urinary bladder
(d) Kidney yin

(s) Large intestine
(d) Lung

(s) Stomach
(d) Spleen/pancreas

(s) Kidney yang
(d) Pericardium

(s) = Superficial
(d) = Deep

Traditional Chinese Treatments: Restoring Balance and Flow.

Since an individual's combinations of yin and yang are unique, TCM practitioners must tailor their treatment to each client. The goal of treatment is to reestablish a balanced flow of energy in the person through diet, herbs, massage, acupuncture, and *Qigong*, a Chinese form of Yoga.

Diet

The simplest and most accessible treatment is diet. Dietary interventions are individualized on the basis of the individual's pattern of disharmony. Foods are used to rebalance the body's internal "climate" by bringing warmth to coldness or cooling off too much heat—that is, by balancing yin and yang. The thermal nature of food is described by the way a person feels after ingesting it. A diet to maintain health should be varied and include a minimum of seven different fruits and vegetables a day to avoid a cold or hot imbalance. If a person is ill and the symptoms indicate a hot condition, then the diet should emphasize cooling foods, and vice versa.

Each food has both yin and yang energies but often one is dominant. Cooling foods and those with bitter and salty flavors are yin. Warming foods are yang, as are foods with pungent and sweet flavors. When people have an excess of yin they may be sluggish, laid back, calm, slightly overweight, and emotionally sensitive. To balance these overly yin tendencies, yang foods are added to the diet to help activate the metabolism and provide more energy. People experiencing an excess of yang may be tense, loud, hyperactive, and aggressive. By adding yin foods to their diets, internal tension can be cooled. See Table 3.2 for a list of common foods and their thermal effects on the body.

Table 3.2   Thermal Properties of Some Common Foods

Cooling	Pork, duck, eggs, clams, crab, millet, barley, wheat, lettuce, celery, broccoli, spinach, tomato, banana, watermelon, asparagus, ice cream, soy sauce
Neutral	Beef, beef liver, rabbit, sardines, yam, rice, corn, rye, potato, beet, turnip, carrot, lemon, apple
Warming	Tuna, turkey, salmon, lamb, venison, chicken, chicken liver, shrimp, trout, oats, cabbage, squash, kale, scallion, celery, ginger, sugar, garlic, pepper

TCM practitioners recommend certain foods for balancing and improving a variety of conditions. Foods can be potent healers, especially when dealing with temporary illnesses, but they are never used as a lone treatment for serious or chronic conditions.

Herbs

Herbal medicine (*ahong yao*) is an integral part of TCM. In terms of the complexity of diagnosis and treatment, it resembles the practice of Western internal medicine. Herbs may be used whole, typically as a tea, or they may be powdered and made into pills, poultices, or tinctures for internal or external use. Just as in food, some herbs are warming (cinnamon) and some are cooling (mint).

With the exception of conditions that require surgery, herbs can be used to treat almost any condition in the practice of TCM. Herbs are often prescribed in complex mixtures and tend not to be used as isolated components, such as extractions from the parent plant. TCM practitioners believe that the healing benefits of herbs result from the synergistic interactions of all the components of the plant. The same herb can be used for many different disorders. Likewise, the same disorder in different people will be treated with different herbs, depending on the practitioner's assessment of the individual. Herbs are used in the following ways: antiviral, antibacterial, antifungal, and anticancer. Herbs are also used to treat pain, aid digestion, lower cholesterol, treat colds and flu, increase resistance to disease, enhance immune function, improve circulation, regulate menstruation, and increase energy. Table 3.3 lists herbs commonly used as tonics in TCM, and Chapter 6, "Herbal Medicine," covers the use of herbs in greater detail.

Table 3.3   Tonic Herbs Frequently Used in TCM

Herb	Use
Garlic	Lowers blood pressure, lowers cholesterol and triglycerides, antiseptic, antifungal
Ginger	Warming effect, stimulates digestion, decreases nausea, relieves aches and pains
Green tea	Lowers cholesterol, anticancer effects, antibacterial effects
Astragalus	Enhances immune function by increasing activity of white blood cells and increases production of antibodies and interferon
Siberian Ginseng	Enhances immune function, increases energy
Ginseng	Increases appetite and digestion, tones skin and muscles, restores depleted sexual energy
Dong Quai (or Tang Kuei)	Blood-building tonic which improves circulation, tones the uterus, balances female hormones
Ho Shou Wu (or Fo Ti)	Cleans the blood, nourishes hair and teeth, increases energy, powerful sexual tonic

Massage

Traditional Chinese massage methods were described in texts as early as 200 BC. Both energizing and sedating massage techniques are used to treat and relieve many medical conditions.

Widely varying illnesses treated with traditional Chinese massage include the common cold, insomnia, leg cramps, painful menses, diarrhea, abdominal pains, headache, asthma, rheumatic pains, stiff neck, colic, nasal bleeding, and throat pains. Massage increases circulation of blood and lymph to the skin and underlying muscles, bringing added nutrients and pain relief. Massage can help restore proper movement to injured limbs and joints and help restore a sense of balance. Massage is an effective method of reducing stress and tension that usually leads to a feeling of relaxation. Chapter 11 covers massage therapy in greater detail.

Acupuncture

Acupuncture involves stimulating specific anatomic points called *hsueh* where each meridian passes close to the skin surface. The primary goal of acupuncture is the manipulation of energy flow throughout the body following a thorough assessment by a TCM practitioner. Puncturing the skin with very fine needles is the usual method but practitioners may also use pressure (*shiatsu*), friction, suction, heat, or electromagnetic energy to stimulate points. *Moxibustion* is an application of heat from certain burning substances at acupuncture points on the body. Ear acupuncture is a complete system within itself and is quite powerful for balancing the hormones and overall energy of the body.

Treatment is offered in the context of the total person and with the goal of correcting the flow of chi to restore health. Some Western health care practitioners who have learned the techniques of acupuncture miss the broader context and limit their focus to an injured or painful body part. Acupuncture is effective in the treatment of acute and chronic pain and motion disabilities. In addition it can be used for the maladies listed below:

- Respiratory and cardiovascular conditions
- Eye, ear, nose, and throat disorders
- Gastrointestinal problems
- Urogenital conditions
- Skin disorders
- Psychiatric problems
- Addictive disorders and withdrawal syndromes.

Chapter 12, "Pressure-Point Therapies," covers acupuncture in more detail.

Qigong

Qigong, pronounced chee-gong, is the art and science of using breath, movement, self-massage, and meditation to cleanse, strengthen, and circulate vital life energy and blood. In India the comparable practice is called *yoga*. Both of these traditions of self-healing have been called "moving meditation" or "meditation in motion." *T'ai Chi*, which is familiar to many Americans, is a more physical form of qigong. In China, millions of people from children to workers, to elders, to patients in the hospital practice qigong daily. The techniques are easy to learn and simple to apply for people who are well or sick. Qigong decreases fatigue and forgetfulness and generates energy by enhancing bodily functions.

caution

People who are pregnant, hemophylic, or who suffer from acute cardiovascular disorders should NOT receive acupuncture treatment.

It is inevitable that taking a deep breath triggers a sense of relaxation. By adding the intention to relax with breathing, the effect is even greater. Adding gentle movements or self-massage to deep breathing and relaxation generates increased self-healing abilities. The focus on deep and intentional relaxation allows for the release of emotional stress, for a sense of tranquility, and for one's natural spirituality to arise.

How Can I Get Started With Traditional Chinese Medicine?

In the 19th century, when large numbers of Chinese laborers arrived in the United States, the immigrant community also included TCM physicians and herbal merchants. Ah Fong Chuck became the first licensed practitioner of TCM in the United States in 1901 when he was awarded a medical license in Idaho. With the advent of World War II and the interruption of the herb supply from China, these practices disappeared or retreated into Chinatowns nationwide. In the 1970s, President Nixon reopened communication with China and the practice of TCM began to gain visibility once again throughout the United States. Now, a clear interest in acupuncture, herbs, and qigong can be found among many North American people. The National Center for Complementary and Alternative Medicine at the NIH is sponsoring many research programs studying the applicability of TCM to common western ailments (see Table 3.4). Their Web site (nccam.nih.gov) is a great place to start an investigation of what kind of TCM might be right for you.

Table 3.4   Studies Funded by the Office of Alternative Medicine at the National Institutes of Health

Medical Condition	TCM Treatment
Unipolar depression	Acupuncture
Osteoarthritis	Acupuncture
Premenstrual syndrome	Traditional Chinese Medicine
Common warts	Chinese herbal therapy
Balance disorders	T'ai Chi
Menopausal hot flashes	Chinese herbal therapy
Postoperative oral surgery pain	Acupuncture
Breech version	Acupuncture
Chronic sinusitis in HIV infection	Traditional Chinese Medicine
Hyperactivity	Acupuncture
Intractable reflex sympathetic Dystrophy	Qigong

Diet

Diet is a primary area where TCM can provide us with some practical guidelines. North Americans seem to have diets of extremes, with fluctuation between overindulgence in food and starvation diets. It is often an all-or-none attitude that has neglected the principle of balance. Limiting the diet to a few fruits and vegetables may be as harmful as a steady diet of hamburgers. In TCM it is believed that illness can be avoided by eating a varied diet as much as possible. For example, avoiding a cold or hot imbalance is accomplished by eating a minimum of seven different fruits and vegetables each day.

For mild, temporary illnesses one might use a number of diet remedies. The cold type of the common cold and flu previously described as characterized by low-grade fever, no sweating, headache, muscle aches, stuffy nose, and a cough with clear white phlegm is treated with warming foods such as garlic, ginger, chives, pepper, pumpkin, apple, onion, and lamb. The hot type of the common cold and flu with its symptoms of high fever, sweating, headache, dry or sore throat, thirst, nasal congestion, and sticky or yellow mucus responds to cooling foods such as watermelon, eggplant, banana, plums, tomato, and tofu.

The cold type of low back pain characterized by coldness and severe pain in the lower back that gradually worsens over time, is not relieved by lying down, and is aggravated by rainy days is treated with hot foods including garlic, chicken, apple, yam, celery, onion, peach, and mustard greens. The hot type of back pain that includes symptoms such as soreness of the lower back that is relieved by lying down, weakness of the legs, and frequent relapses is treated with cooling foods such as peanuts, sesame, soybeans, beef, pineapple, and grapes.

Breathing and Relaxation

Like many other forms of alternative therapies, TCM regards breath as an important function of life. Restrictions in breathing lead to dysfunction and disease. Forming healthy breathing habits can counter stress and help balance body, mind, emotions, and spirit.

Throughout the day one may find hundreds of opportunities to integrate some deep breathing, relaxation, self-massage, and gentle movement techniques into usual activities. For example, you could try any one of these techniques:

- You are sitting at a stoplight. Take a deep breath.
- You are just about to fall asleep or have just awakened. Breathe deeply and allow your whole body to become completely relaxed.
- You are in the shower washing your hair. As you apply shampoo, massage your scalp vigorously; rub your ears, relax, take several deep breaths.
- As you apply lotion or oil to your body following your bath, do so with the intent of relaxing each muscle group as you gently massage your entire body.
- You are watching television. During each commercial break, massage your hands, feet, and ears. Breathe deeply and relax.
- You are vacuuming the house. Relax your shoulders, breathe deeply, and coordinate your movements with your breathing.

THE ABSOLUTE MINIMUM

- Traditional Chinese Medicine is primarily concerned with the detection and correction of imbalances within and around the body.
- TCM uses diet, breathing, acupuncture, and herbal treatments to correct imbalances.
- In China, TCM techniques are practiced alongside, and often integrated with, Western biomedical techniques.

RESOURCES

- Council of Colleges of Acupuncture and Oriental Medicine

  www.ccaom.org

- Academy of Chinese Culture and Health Science

  www.acchs.edu

- American Academy of Medical Acupuncture

  www.medicalacupuncture.org

- Cathay Herbal Laboratories

  www.cathayherbal.com

4

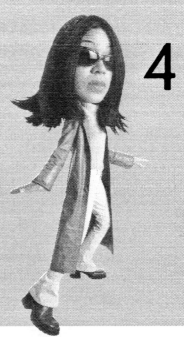

Ayurvedic Medicine

Ayurveda, one of the oldest medical systems in the world, has been practiced for 4,000 years in India. It is a holistic and sophisticated system encompassing the balance of body, mind, and spirit as well as balance among people, their environments, and the larger cosmos. Ayurveda is a Sanskrit word derived from two roots—*ayur*, which means life, and *veda*, or knowledge—and translates literally to the science of life. Ayurveda has been adapted by Hindu, Buddhist, and other religious groups and is undergoing a renaissance both in India and throughout the West.

Ayurveda is an intricate system with a tradition of integrating useful concepts and practices from other systems. This ancient system has adapted to modern science and technology, including biomedical science and quantum physics. In this blending, Ayurveda and conventional medicine have been completely compatible.

What Is Ayurveda?

Ayurveda asserts a fundamental connection between the microcosm and macrocosm. People are a creation of the cosmos and as such are minute representations of the universe, containing within them everything that makes up the surrounding world. One must understand the world in order to understand people and, conversely, understand people in order to understand the world. Ayurveda emphasizes the interdependence of the health of the individual and the quality of societal life. Therefore, measures to ensure the collective health of society, such as pollution control and appropriate living conditions, are encouraged.

The Five Elements

Ayurveda views nature and people as made up of five elements or qualities. These elements are earth, water, fire, air, and space; they are believed to be composed of both matter and energy. As the elements interact, they give rise to all that exists:

- The earth element is dense, heavy, and hard. In the human body, all solid structures and compact tissues are derived from the earth element.

- The water element is liquid and soft and exists in many forms in the body such as plasma, cytoplasm, saliva, nasal secretion, eye secretion, and cerebrospinal fluid.

- The fire element is hot and light and is believed to regulate body temperature as well as being responsible for digestion, absorption, and assimilation. The solar plexus is the seat of fire in the body. Fire manifests in the brain as the gray matter that allows one to recognize, appreciate, and comprehend the world.

- The air element is cold, mobile, and rough, and in the cosmos is the magnetic field responsible for the movement of the earth, wind, and water. In the body, the air element governs cellular function, the movement of breath, and movements of the intestines. Thought, desire, and will are also governed by the air principle.

- The space element is clear and subtle and makes up most of our bodies. Space plays a unique role because it allows the existence of sound, which needs space in order to travel. Sound includes not only audible sound like music but subtler vibrations that resonate in our bodies.

People are a composite of these five elements, which combine in various ways to govern mind, body, and spirit. Ayurveda sees the body functioning through the interaction of three systems: *doshas* (vital energies), *dhatus* (tissues), and *malas* (waste products). The vital energy controls the creation of all the various tissues of the body and effects the removal of unnecessary waste products from the body.

Doshas

Doshas are both structures and energy; they are the mediators between body tissues, wastes, and the environment. They are responsible for all physiological and psychological processes. The Sanskrit names for the three doshas are *Vata*, *Pitta*, and *Kapha*. As the driver or mover of the entire body, the Vata dosha is the most important. It is composed of the elements of air and space and is involved with all elimination, physical and mental movement, and nervous function. If Vata becomes imbalanced, it can cause the other two doshas to become imbalanced. The Pitta dosha is composed of the elements fire and water, governs enzymes and hormones, and is responsible for digestion, body temperature, hunger, thirst, sight, complexion, courage, and mental activity. The Kapha dosha, composed of the elements of earth and water, is the heaviest of the three doshas. It provides the structure, strength, and stability that the body needs. It is also responsible for lubrication, sexual power, and fertility. Figure 4.1 illustrates the connections between the elements and the doshas.

FIGURE 4.1

A Framework for Nature: The Elements and the Doshas.

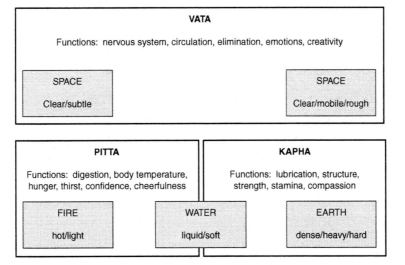

Body Types

Vata, Pitta, and Kapha are present in every cell, tissue, and organ, but each person is made up of unique ratios of the three doshas. This individual constitution is determined by genetics, diet, lifestyle, and emotions.

The basic pattern of the Vata type is "changeable." Vata people are unpredictable and often start things without finishing them. Stress usually leads to anxiety or fear. They are responsive to sound and touch and dislike loud noise. Balanced Vata people are happy, enthusiastic, and energetic. When out of balance they have a tendency to be impulsive.

The basic pattern of the Pitta type is "intense." Pitta people are ambitious, outspoken, bold, orderly, and efficient. They tend to respond to the world visually and enjoy being surrounded by fine objects. Balanced Pitta people are sweet, joyous, and confident.

The basic pattern of the Kapha type is "relaxed." Kapha people are stable, steady people who have a happy, tranquil view of the world. They are graceful people who wake up slowly, eat slowly, and speak slowly. They respond to the world through taste and smell and tend to place a great deal of importance on food.

More detailed descriptions of the dosha types, as well as guidance in determining your dosha type, can be found later in this chapter.

Dosha Composites

According to Ayurveda, the three doshas may appear in different combinations in different people, resulting in ten composite body types, as shown in Table 4.1. Knowing one's body type is the key to balancing one's life in the way that nature intended. This balance goes beyond physical and mental health and includes personal relationships, work satisfaction, spiritual growth, and social harmony. As a general rule, the strongest dosha in one's constitution has the greatest tendency to increase, making people most susceptible to illnesses associated with an increase of that dosha.

Table 4.1   Dosha Combinations Result in Distinct Body Types

- Single dosha types: One dosha is predominant
  Vata
  Pitta
  Kapha

- Two-dosha types: One dosha is predominant with a strong secondary dosha
  Vata-Pitta, Pitta-Vata
  Pitta-Kapha, Kapha-Pitta
  Kapha-Vata, Vata-Kapha

- Three-dosha type: All three doshas are in equal proportions
  Vata-Pitta-Kapha

Few people are single-dosha types. Most are two-dosha types, with one dosha predominant but not extreme. The dominant dosha gives people their primary reactions to the world, which are then moderated by the second dosha.

Those with the two doshas of Vata-Pitta type are quick-moving, friendly, and talkative with a sharp intellect. They are not as unpredictable or irregular as the single Vata type. They enjoy challenges but stress makes them tense and hard-driven.

People who have a combination of Pitta and Kapha types are stable personalities but have a tendency toward anger and criticism. They have steady energy and good stamina but are less motivated to be active.

Those whose doshas are the Kapha and Vata type may have a hard time identifying themselves since the Vata and Kapha tend to be opposites. Usually they have a thin body type but with a relaxed, easygoing manner. They tend to procrastinate but can be quick and efficient when necessary. The three-dosha type tends to have good immunity, lifelong good health, and longevity.

Tissues/*Dhatus*

The seven *dhatus* or tissues are the structures of the body responsible for nourishment, and must be retained for health. They are *rasa* (plasma), *rakta* (blood cells), *mamsa* (muscle), *meda* (fat), *asthi* (bone), *majja* (bone marrow), and *shukra* (reproductive tissue). In general, Ayurveda practitioners work to keep these tissues intact and healthy.

Waste Products/*Malas*

The *malas*, or wastes, are the nonretainable substances within the body. Urine, feces, and sweat, for example, need to be released and eliminated as the body rids itself of toxins. Excreting the *malas* cleanses, so Ayurveda advises not to inhibit the body's natural functions, including sneezing, yawning, burping, urinating, defecating, and passing gases. Vata is the dosha that causes these urges, and suppression of them disturbs Vata. Ayurveda does encourage expression of these urges in a way that is not offensive to other people.

Energy/*Prana*

Prana, which the Chinese call *chi*, in Sanskrit means "primary energy," sometimes translated as "breath" or "vital force." Prana is not only the basic life force, it is the original creative power. Prana has many levels of meaning, from the physical breath to the energy of consciousness. The five pranas are categorized according to movement, direction, and body region. The navel is considered the pranic center of the physical body.

Balancing the Doshas: The Ayurvedic View of Health and Illness

Ayurvedic practitioners regard the balance of the doshas as their primary diagnostic indicator. When the doshas are balanced, individuals experience health on all levels: mental, emotional, physical, and spiritual. It is much more than the mere absence of disease. Mentally healthy people have good memory, comprehension, intelligence, and reasoning ability. Emotionally healthy people experience evenly balanced emotional states and a sense of well-being or happiness. Physically healthy people have abundant energy with proper functioning of the senses, digestion, and elimination. Spiritually healthy people have a sense of aliveness and richness in life, are developing in the direction of their full potential, and are in good relationship with themselves, other people, and the larger cosmos.

Balancing one's doshas does not mean trying to achieve an equal portion of Vata, Pita, and Kapha. One cannot change the ratio of doshas that are present from conception. Health is the balance of each dosha that is right for that particular individual. Doshas, however, are responsive to people's habits, such as diet, exercise, and daily routines, which can either deplete or increase the doshas. While both states of imbalance lead to ill-health or disease, increased doshas are more problematic than decreased doshas.

Imbalance in the doshas is the first sign that mind, body, and spirit are not perfectly coordinated. One type, called natural imbalance, is due to time and age. Natural imbalances are typically mild and normally do not cause problems. Each dosha becomes more predominant during certain times of day, as energy moves through six cycles in each 24-hour period: Veta predominates from 2 to 6, day and night; Kapha during the hours of 6 to 10; and Pita from 10 until 2. Each dosha also predominates during particular seasons and stages of life. Kapha is predominate during childhood and during the spring season, Pita during summer and middle age, and Vata during fall and the latter part of one's life.

Unnatural balances of the doshas can be caused by a variety of factors, each of which falls into one of three broad categories of disease. *Adhyatmika* diseases originate within the body and include hereditary and congenital diseases. *Adhibhautika* diseases originate outside the body and include trauma, bacteria, and viruses. *Adhidaivika* diseases originate from supernatural sources, including those diseases that are otherwise unexplainable, such as illnesses originating from seasonal changes, divine sources, planetary influences, and curses. While some of these causes are beyond individual control, lifestyle and diet are within one's control. Preventing disease and improving overall health depends on the recognition of dosha imbalance and an understanding of the factors that increase and decrease each of the doshas.

Imbalanced Vata shows up as rough skin, weight loss, anxiety, restlessness, insomnia, decreased strength, constipation, arthritis, hypertension, rheumatic disorder, and cardiac arrhythmia. Pita imbalance includes a yellowish complexion, excessive body heat, insufficient sleep, weak digestion, inflammation, inflammatory bowel disease, skin disease, heartburn, and peptic ulcer. Kapha imbalance presents as a pale complexion, coldness, lethargy, excessive sleep, depression, sinusitis, respiratory disease, asthma, and excessive weight gain.

A number of factors aggravate or increase each of the doshas. Factors increasing Vata are excessive exercise, wakefulness, falling, cold, late autumn and winter, fear or grief, agitation or anger, fasting, and pungent, astringent, bitter foods. Factors increasing Pita are anger, fasting, strong sunshine, midsummer and early autumn, and pungent, sour, or salty food. Kapha is increased by factors such as sleeping during the daytime, spring and early summer, heavy food, mild products, sugar, and sweet, sour, or salty foods.

How Does Ayurveda Work?

The first question an Ayurvedic practitioner asks is not "What disease does this person have?" but "Who is this person?" The complete process of diagnosis takes into account physical, mental, and spiritual components integrated with the social and environmental worlds in which the person lives. In addition to using x-rays or other biomedical diagnostic tools, Ayurvedic practitioners diagnose by observing people, touching them, taking pulses, and interviewing them.

Ayurvedic Diagnosis: The Whole Body Tells the Story

Pulse diagnosis is a highly specialized skill that requires great sensitivity. The process involves placing the index, middle, and ring fingers of the right hand on the radial arteries of the right hand of men and the left hand of women. Pulse diagnosis is remarkably comprehensive. Experienced physicians can not only diagnose present diseases but can also tell what diseases the person has experienced in the past and which are likely to develop in the future.

Tongue diagnosis can also reveal the functional status of internal organs. A healthy tongue should be pink, clear, and shiny. A discoloration and/or sensitivity of a particular area of the tongue indicates dosha dysfunction. Kapha imbalance is evidenced by a whitish tongue, Pitta imbalance a yellow-green tongue, and Vata imbalance a brown to black tongue.

Ayurvedic practitioners do urine examinations as another way to understand dosha imbalances. A midstream specimen is collected first thing in the morning. Healthy urine should be clear without much foam. Kapha imbalance gives the urine a cloudy appearance, Pitta imbalance imparts a dark yellow color, and pale yellow and oily urine indicates a Vata imbalance. The practitioner also puts a few drops of sesame oil in the urine and examines it in the sunlight. The shape of the drops signifies which dosha is imbalanced: a snake-like shape with wave movement indicates Vata, an umbrella shape with multiple colors, Pitta, and a pearl shape, Kapha. The movement of the oil in the urine indicates the prognosis of the disease. If the drop spreads immediately, the illness is probably easy to cure. If the oil drops to the middle of the urine sample, the illness is more difficult to cure. If the oil sinks to the bottom, the illness may be impossible to cure.

The practitioner also carefully examines the skin, nails, and lips. Cool, hot, rough or dry skin indicate imbalance. Imbalance can be visualized in the nails by longitudinal striations, bumps, or a parrot beak at the end of the nail. Dry, rough lips or inflammatory patches on the lips are another sign of imbalance. Coldness, dryness, roughness, and cracking indicate Vata imbalance. Hotness and redness indicate Pitta imbalance. Kapha imbalance is indicated by wetness, whiteness, and coldness.

Ayurvedic Treatments Will Change Your Life

Specific lifestyle interventions are a major preventive and therapeutic approach in Ayurveda. Each person is prescribed an individualized diet and exercise program depending on dosha type and the nature of the underlying dosha imbalance. Herbal preparations are added to the diet for preventive or regenerative purposes as well as for the treatment of specific disorders. Practitioners also prescribe Yoga, breathing exercises, and meditative techniques.

Nutrition

In Ayurveda, a balanced diet is different from the Western perspective of a balanced diet derived from the basic food groups of meat, dairy, fruit, grains, and vegetables. Ayurveda recognizes six tastes: sweet, sour, salty, pungent, bitter, and astringent. A balanced Ayurveda diet must contain all six tastes at every meal but in different proportions depending on dosha type. The word "taste" includes not only the perceptions on the tongue but also the immediate effect of the substances within the body. Each of the six tastes is derived from two of the five elements as illustrated in Figure 4.2. Sour, salty, and pungent have the fire element and so increase body temperature, dilate body channels, and allow energy and toxins to flow out from the body. Sweet, bitter, and astringent have no fire and thus are cooling, promoting relaxation. Sweet, sour, and salty have the water element and soften tissues, lubricate mucus membranes, and increase water retention.

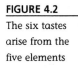

FIGURE 4.2

The six tastes arise from the five elements

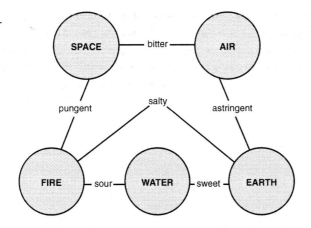

It is not necessary to memorize which foods carry which tastes or reduce which doshas, as there are any number of books offering long lists of food doshas and tastes. Many people seem to know naturally what their bodies need for balance. See Table 4.2 for the relationship between the doshas and tastes, and for some foods that will reduce an excess of each dosha.

Table 4.2   Foods in Relation to Doshas

Dosha	Balanced by	Aggravated by	To Reduce, Eat
Vata	Salt, Sour, Sweet	Pungent, Bitter, Astringent	Asparagus, carrots, green beans, avocados, bananas, melons, rice, wheat, chicken, seafood, chickpeas, and tofu
Pitta	Bitter, Sweet, Astringent	Pungent, Sour, Salty	Broccoli, cabbage, lettuce, apples, grapes, raisins, barley, oats, ice cream, chicken, shrimp, chickpeas, tofu, and coconut, olive, and soy oils
Kapha	Pungent, Bitter, Astringent	Sweet, Sour, Salty	Cauliflower, celery, leafy green vegetables, apricots, pears, dried fruits in general, barley, corn, rye, skim milk, chicken, shrimp, sunflower seeds, and raw honey

To counter an excess of Vata, diet recommendations consist of warm food with moderately heavy textures, salt, sour, and sweet tastes, and added oil. To counter an excess of Pitta, diet recommendations are for cool or warm (but not hot) foods with moderately heavy textures and bitter, sweet, and astringent tastes. For an excess of Kapha, diet recommendations include warm, light food, cooked without much water; pungent, bitter, and astringent tastes; and a minimum of butter and oil. The goal of diet management is to achieve the balance of tastes that, for you, will avoid aggravating any of the doshas and keep them calm and balanced.

Herbs

In Ayuveda, natural medicines are primarily herbal but may include animal and mineral ingredients, and even powdered gemstones. Practitioners prescribe thousands of herbs. Like food, herbs are classified according to the six tastes. Herbs, however, are more potent and specific in their action than food. Some herbs, used for preventive and regenerative purposes, are readily available. The use of herbs for treating disease must be medically supervised. As in Traditional Chinese Medicine, the entire plant is used. It is believed that the plant contains other chemicals that buffer the active ingredient, thus reducing possible side effects.

Like foods, herbs balance doshas. Vata balancing herbs include ginseng, licorice, Indian Pennywort, Bala, and Sitopladi. Pitta dosha is balanced by aloe vera, comfrey root, Indian Gooseberry, and saffron; Kapha dosha by elecampane, honey, and sitopladi balancing. Herbs usually take longer to work than Western medications prescribed by practitioners.

Historically, Ayurvedic herbs have had little exposure outside India but are now becoming more familiar, and available, with the rapid explosion of herbal medicine in North America. Sitopladi is a very good herbal formula for colds and flu. Indian Pennywort (*brahmi*) enhances a person's ability to focus mentally and learn new material. Guggulu is a powerful purifying agent, well known for lowering of blood cholesterol levels. Shilajit, with its antispasmodic qualities, is effective in acute and chronic respiratory illnesses. Bala, or Indian Country Mallow, is helpful in all types of nervous system disorders and certain types of heart disease. These few examples of herbs give one an idea of how they are used as natural body medicines. Chapter 6, "Herbal Medicine," presents herbs in more detail. Numerous books on the market and various Web sites describe the use of herbs in alternative medicine.

Exercise

According to Ayurveda, exercise should conform to one's dosha type. Kapha people can perform moderately heavy exercise such as aerobics, running, dancing, and weight training. Because of their physical strength, Kaphas excel at endurance sports. Pitta people, who have more drive than endurance and an intense competitive spirit, should have a moderate amount of exercise. Brisk walking or jogging, hiking, swimming, and skiing are appropriate. People with a Vata dosha might enjoy jogging, but exercises like stretching, yoga, and T'ai Chi are better choices. They have bursts of energy but tire quickly and may push themselves past their limits. Walking is probably the best exercise for all people as it calms all dosha types. Ayurveda recommends a brisk half-hour walk every day.

For people over the age of 80 or under 10 as well as those people who have serious Vata and Pitta imbalance, exercise should be very gentle. Exercise should always leave a person ready for work as opposed to exercise being work itself. Several other exercise precautions must be noted. One should not engage in exercise sooner than half an hour before and one to two hours after a meal. Exercising in the evening is discouraged because it is better for the body to slow down and prepare for sleep. Exercise is discouraged in the wind or cold since heavy breathing of cold, damp air is unhealthy for the respiratory tract. Also discouraged is exercise during the intense heat of the day, since environmental heat causes an even greater rise in body temperature.

The key to exercise is moderation and regularity. Ayurveda suggests that all exercise should be done at one-half of one's capacity. That means working out just until sweat appears on the forehead, under the arms, and along the spinal column. This amount of exercise improves digestion, prevents constipation, improves circulation, stimulates metabolism, regulates body temperature, and maintains body weight. Exercise keeps one's senses and mind alert and attentive as well as being effective in inducing relaxation and sleep. Overexercise, as indicated by panting and heavy sweating, may cause dehydration, muscle aches, breathlessness, and even chest pain. It is believed that overexercise eventually contributes to arthritis, sciatica, or heart conditions.

Yoga, developed in the Ayurvedic tradition, is one of the most effective forms of exercise for the body as well as nourishment for the mind and spirit. Hatha yoga, the most familiar form of yoga in North America, is a combination of body positions, breathing exercises, and mental focus on the here-and-now. Stretching helps relax and tone the muscles, improves circulation and concentration, and helps reenergize. Yoga is increasingly recognized for maintaining general health as well as helping people to manage chronic disorders such as headaches, insomnia, hypertension, and depression. Further information about yoga can be found in Chapter 15.

Breathing

Practicing controlled breathing is a valuable technique that leads to a healthier lifestyle. Several techniques can be utilized to relax the mind and body. Simple breathing helps people become aware of their breath and often relieves tension.

Simple breathing involves closing the eyes and observing the breath, becoming more aware of its pattern and changes. Slow, easy breathing is continued for several minutes until a sense of relaxation is achieved.

TRY IT YOURSELF: *PRANAYAMA*

Alternate nostril breathing, *Pranayama*, is another technique that can ease difficulty in breathing by making the respiratory rhythm more regular, which in turn soothes the entire nervous system. Pranayama is helpful prior to meditation because it focuses attention inward. Pranayama is performed while seated with the eyes closed. Figure 4.3 illustrates the position. The index and middle fingers of the right hand are placed in between the eyebrows. The thumb closes the right nostril while the person breathes in through the left nostril. The left nostril is then closed with the ring finger and the right nostril is opened for the out breath and the next in breath. The right nostril is then closed and the out breath occurs through the left nostril. After doing a couple of rounds, breathing naturally gets deeper and smoother.

FIGURE 4.3

Many experience less tension and increased relaxation by focusing on controlled breathing exercises.

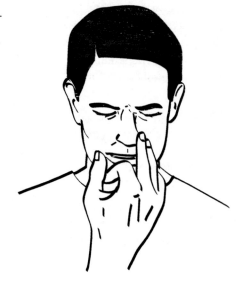

Meditation

An important part of daily life in Ayurveda, meditation is considered a powerful tool to help maintain health. Meditation is a moment-to-moment awareness that is cleansing to the body, mind, and spirit. It is finding the quiet in the mind. As the mind is brought into a silent and receptive state, new energy comes into being, which is conducive to a state of health and peace. Further information about meditation can be found in Chapter 16.

Massage

Marma therapy is a massage technique focusing on 107 sensitive points, called marmas, located on the skin. These points are similar to the acupuncture points called hsueh in Traditional Chinese Medicine. Marma therapy predates the Chinese approach and is likely the parent to acupuncture and acupressure. Marmas are activated through various methods. One is through yoga movements that gently stretch specific marma points. Warm oil dripped on the center of the forehead, a major marma point, can be profoundly soothing. A daily self-massage with oil can reach all the marmas on the skin, and can be found, along with further information on massage, in Chapter 11.

Aromatherapy

Aromatherapy is based on olfactory stimuli used to help balance the doshas as each responds to specific signals. Specialized olfactory cells provide instant connection of odors with the brain. The hypothalamus responds through regulation of bodily functions, the limbic system responds with emotions, and the hippocampus responds with memories, which explains how smells can elicit memories so vividly.

In general, Vata is balanced with warm, sweet, and sour aromas such as basil, orange, rose geranium, clove, and other spices. Pitta is balanced by sweet, cool aromas such as rose, mint, cinnamon, sandalwood, and jasmine. Kapha is balanced using warm aromas with spicy overtones such as juniper, eucalyptus, camphor, and clove. People whose doshas are out of balance are given specific oils to restore dosha balance. Aromatherapy may be used at any time but is often prescribed at night as it helps induce sleep. Aromatherapy is discussed further in Chapter 9.

Music

India has a long tradition of merging music and medicine. Unlike most Western music in which the notes are distinct, the tones tend to blend together, creating a soothing, unifying sound. As with taste and smell, doshas can be balanced with certain tones and rhythms. The three doshas peak at different times of the day and traditional Indian music smoothes the process of these transitions. An example of a rough transition is the inability to fall asleep because one's mind is racing with many thoughts. Ten minutes of music can be used as a gentle wakeup in the morning, after a meal to settle digestion, just before bedtime to aid sleep, and during the recovery period from an illness.

Purification

Panchakarma, or purification therapy, involves five procedures, any or all of which can be chosen based on the person's general condition, the season, and the nature of the disease. The five therapies of Panchakarma are experienced over a period of a week and involve purifying the body through the use of sweating, emetics, purgatives, enemas, and nasal inhalations. Commonly administered by an Ayurvedic physician with the help of a number of assistants, the benefits of Panchakarma are relief from long-standing symptoms, renewed health, and extended longevity.

How Can I Get Started with Ayurveda?

Since Ayurveda is a comprehensive philosophy of health, you can begin an Ayurvedic practice by thinking about therapies you may already be using (herbal medicine, massage, aromatherapy) within the context of Ayurvedic thought. If you find that taking an Ayurvedic outlook has positively affected your feelings of health, you can deepen your involvement in the philosophy of Ayurveda. The resources section of this chapter is a great places to start such an investigation.

Determining Your Dosha

The first step to adopting an Ayurvedic perspective on your health is to determine your dosha type. See Table 4.3 for the checklist and follow these steps to determine dosha type:

- Make a check mark next to the description that best describes how you have been most of your life. If you fall between two descriptions, check both of them.

- Consider the qualities carefully. There are no right or wrong answers. Be honest and check how you are, not how you would like to be.

- Look for lasting trends. For example, if your sleep has been heavy and for long periods of time most of your life but you are now sleeping light and fitfully, the change is likely to be due to imbalance rather than dosha type. Check your usual pattern.

- Notice whether each dosha has some checks, because everyone has Vata, Pitta, and Kapha as part of their body type.

- Total the number of checks for each dosha. The dosha with the greatest number should be your body type. If the highest two doshas are close, you are probably a two-dosha type. If all three dosha scores are close, you have a three dosha type.

Table 4.3 Your Dosha Checklist

Vata Dosha	Pitta Dosha	Kapha Dosha
❏ light, thin build	❏ medium build	❏ solid, powerful build
❏ thin, dry skin	❏ fair, soft, warm skin	❏ thick, pale, cold, oily, smooth skin
❏ dark, coarse, curly hair	❏ fine, soft, blond, light brown or red hair	❏ thick, wavy, lustrous hair
❏ irregular hunger and digestion, tendency toward constipation	❏ sharp hunger and thirst, strong digestion, cannot skip meals	❏ slow digestion, mild hunger
❏ difficulty putting on weight	❏ no problem gaining or losing weight	❏ tendency to obesity, hard to lose weight
❏ light, interrupted sleep	❏ sleep is sound but short	❏ sleep is heavy and for long period of time
❏ aversion to cold weather, craves warmth	❏ aversion to hot weather, craves coolness	❏ aversion to cold, damp weather
❏ bursts of mental and physical energy	❏ moderate strength and endurance	❏ steady energy, great strength and endurance
❏ performs activity quickly	❏ aggressive and competitive in physical activity	❏ graceful in action
❏ quick to grasp new information, also quick to forget	❏ sharp intellect, good, quick memory	❏ slow to grasp new information, good retentive memory
❏ tendency for worry, anxiety, fearfulness	❏ tendency toward anger, irritability under stress, judgmental	❏ tendency to be complacent, greedy, possessive
❏ excitability, changing moods	❏ busy lifestyle, achiever	❏ affectionate, tolerant, forgiving
❏ enthusiasm, vivaciousness	❏ enterprising character, likes challenges	❏ good organizer
❏ fast talking	❏ speech is sharp, clear, precise	❏ speech is slow, may be labored
❏ illnesses: degenerative, related to being underweight, or those interfering with movement	❏ illnesses: inflammation, bleeding	❏ illnesses: swellings, tumors, those related to overweight
Vata Total	Pitta Total	Kapha Total

Determining dosha type allows you to begin to understand how your health is affected by internal and external influences as you consider your unique blend of doshas. As you become more familiar with your body, you can observe and experience the effect of what you eat and do each day, how you think and feel, the state of your metabolism, digestion, and elimination, the relationships you engage in, your jobs, and the environment in which you find yourself. Because all of these factors are interdependent, problems in one area can cause problems in other areas.

Seeking Dosha Balance

People's dosha balance can be disrupted in a number of ways. An inappropriate diet and lifestyle for your dosha type will cause a slowly developing excess or deficiency in doshas. If you suffer significant trauma, however, the dosha levels can change immediately and dramatically. Dosha imbalance can also occur from an accumulation of toxins or when too many experiences of a particular dosha take place without enough experiences from the other doshas. Once you understand your baseline dosha type, you can assess imbalances that may contribute to disease. Remember, it is the strongest dosha in your constitution that has the greatest tendency to increase.

For example, if you have a Kapha dosha type, you have a natural tendency to those things that have Kapha qualities, thus increasing your Kapha energy. If you have a lifestyle that includes overeating, not exercising, and sleeping excessively, and you have a desk job, your Kapha dosha can become excessive. You may need to consciously add opposite qualities to pacify or balance your Kapha energy such as decrease your food intake, eat more pungent and bitter vegetables and astringent fruits, and increase your exercise.

Achieving balance of the doshas does not happen quickly—you need to work at it consciously. In some cases, lifestyle changes may be difficult, such as the nature of your job, while others may be easier, such as a change in leisure activities. Typically, people find that diet, exercise, and leisure activities are the most amenable to change. For example, television and computers increase Vata through stimulation of the eyes and ears and increase Kapha by the passive nature of these activities. If the television program makes you angry or your computer program will not do what you wish, your Pitta may be stimulated. Limiting the time spent watching television and being selective with programs may help you balance your doshas and move toward a healthier state. Likewise, if you spend a lot of time at your computer, you need to take frequent breaks, move and stretch your body, and rest your eyes.

Balancing Vata Dosha

If your strongest dosha is Vata, you need to develop more regularity in your daily routines such as eating regular meals, having an established bedtime, and slowing down and taking time to think. Because you have a tendency to dry skin, oil your skin regularly.

People with Vata doshas are drawn to sensory experiences involving movement, speed, and action, and you may enjoy loud music and computer games. To maintain a healthy balance, make an effort to balance those activities with quiet, creative pursuits such as writing, photography, or painting. Similarly, because you are attracted to vigorous exercise, try to engage in gentle exercise every day. Remember, Ayurveda suggests that all exercise be done at one-half of one's capacity. If you know that you are exhausted after a 40-minute aerobic class, then you should do only 20 minutes of the class.

People with Vata doshas enjoy spending their vacations sightseeing, touring, and filling their days and nights with many activities and returning home exhausted. A more beneficial vacation would be in a beautiful, sunny, and warm environment where you rest and limit your activities. If you are a Vata type, your clothes are mostly dark shades that may reflect a tendency to become depressed. Bright yellow colors and pastel shades may brighten your mood.

Balancing Pitta Dosha

If you are a Pitta type, you need to loosen up on setting and achieving goals and learn to enjoy here-and-now moments. You can learn to achieve your ambitions without pressuring yourself. Your need to organize yourself, and everyone else, must be kept under control lest you become easily frustrated when things do not go as planned.

You are stimulated by competitive, mentally challenging situations that may increase your aggression or your determination to win. Learn to use constructive criticism rather than confrontation. Engaging in noncompetitive leisure activities such as gardening may help prevent an excess of Pitta.

Vacations in cooler climates and water and winter sports will cool your tendency to be warm. Avoid organizing your vacations in the greatest of detail and try to enjoy whatever happens. Red clothing overstimulates Pitta and may contribute to a more aggressive approach to others. Cool, soft, pale colors are more balancing to the Pitta dosha.

Balancing Kapha Dosha

If you are a Kapha type, you need to vary your daily experiences to avoid becoming stuck in a rut. Try to make small changes in routine every day. Get up early and go to bed late to limit your tendency to sleep many hours.

Since you may prefer to sit and do nothing, find activities that are mentally and physically stimulating. Kapha is balanced by vigorous exercise but you will most likely have to force yourself. Because you have good stamina, you can exercise for a longer time than people who are Vata or Pitta.

You would prefer a vacation lying on a beach doing nothing but soaking up the sun. You will find, however, that sightseeing and touring will be more stimulating and balancing for you. All colors, except greens and dark blues, balance Kapha. You will find that bright, strong colors are exciting and balancing.

Understanding your doshas is an ongoing process. As you observe your mind, body, spirit, and relationships, you will learn how you respond to different qualities in everyday activities. When you're sure what your dosha type is, think about your lifestyle in terms of diet, work, leisure activities, exercise, daily routines, quiet times, sleep, and relationships. Applying the principles of Ayurveda, you can begin making choices about the qualities you want incorporated into your life. Don't focus on negatives—"I shouldn't…"—think about what you want to *start* doing. Then, try to limit your exposure to those qualities you do not want, and spend more time enjoying those that will aid your well-being. Change begins with small steps and is a gradual process. You may want to seek the advice of an Ayurvedic practitioner to individualize a lifestyle change program. Remember: mind and body always strive toward health; with time, nurturing, routine, and gentle discipline, you can achieve a more complete level of well-being.

THE ABSOLUTE MINIMUM

- The Indian health system Ayurveda sees the body functioning through the interaction of vital energies, body tissues, and waste products.
- Ayurveda uses eating practices, herbal treatments, massage, meditation, and postural and breathing exercises to balance the interaction of these three agents and foster the deepest experience of health.
- Knowing one's body type, or dosha, is the first and most important step in adopting an Ayurvedic lifestyle.

RESOURCES

- The Ayurvedic Institute

  www.ayurveda.com
- Ayurvedic Foundations

  www.ayur.com
- Jiva Ayurveda

  www.ayurvedic.org

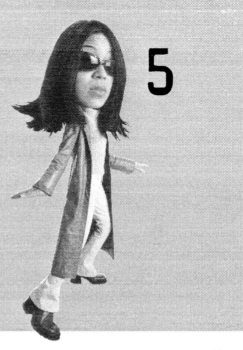

5

NATIVE AMERICAN HEALING

The population of today's Native American tribes is only a fraction of what it was before Europeans invaded this continent. Forty-five percent of all Native Americans living on reservations live below the poverty level, Native Americans have the highest infant mortality rate of any group in the United States, and life expectancy among Native Americans on reservations is under 50 years of age. Many customs have been lost forever. Despite these impediments, many of the traditions and ceremonies practiced by Native Americans for centuries are still in evidence today. Although each Native American Indian-based healing system is unique, they share a number of characteristics. This chapter presents the commonalities found among tribes.

What Is Native American Healing?

Most tribal people have one or more types of healthcare specialists that frequently overlap. Some Native healers use herbs, some heal with songs, and some with spiritual rituals. A midwife or a medicine woman or man might focus on natural medicines such as herbs and hands-on techniques but also use prayer and ceremony. *Shamans* or holy people emphasize spiritual healing but are often also knowledgeable about natural medicines. *Kahunas* are people, usually of Hawaiian ancestry, who have developed a level of spirituality that joins them with many of the spirit powers allowing direct communication about the healing process.

To learn, people must be open to the ancient wisdom and understand it in the context of the entire Native American experience. It is not something to be trivialized by simply purchasing medicine objects and trying them out at home. As one Sioux leader said, "First they took our land, now they want our pipes ... all the wannabees, these New Agers, come with their crystals and want to buy a medicine bag to carry them around in. If you want to learn our ways, come walk the red road with us, but be silent and listen."

The Spiritual Foundation of Native American Medicine

Spirituality and medicine are inseparable in Native American tradition. Essentially no distinction is made between religious and medical practices. "Making medicine" is an important part of traditional life. It is how people give thanks to the Spirit who helps, guides, nourishes, and clothes them. Medicine is the constant pipeline to the Creator. In Native American tradition, making medicine is a process for achieving a variety of positive outcomes: a good hunt, plentiful crops, connecting with someone, healing someone, a successful birthing, and so on. Medicine is the way people keep their balance; it provides them with the opportunity to grow in new and healthier ways

Native Americans believe in a singular living God, but also believe that same God may be contacted in many different ways. In Native languages, God is given such names as Great Spirit, Creator, Great Being, Great Mystery, Above Being, The One Who Oversees All Things, and He Who Gives Life. The missionaries mistakenly thought that Native American people worshiped trees, eagles, the Pipe, and many other things. What was misinterpreted was the use of these objects as gifts from the Creator, put here to help and to serve as conduits to greater understanding of the Creator's ways. Using these gifts is one way to create an atmosphere conducive to addressing the Creator.

Gratitude is a central aspect of Native American culture. Every day is a spiritual, sacred day. One morning prayer, for example, is, "I thank You for another day. I ask that You give me the strength to walk worthily this day so that when I lie down at night I will not be ashamed." Thanks are given to the Great Power who makes all things possible. People give thanks, not only for the good events but also for the bad things that happen throughout the day, because they believe that the more they show their appreciation, the more blessings they will receive.

The Healing Art: a Gift from the Creator

Shamans and medicine people are seen as channels the Creator has provided and trained. Some are born into families with medical or ritual skills, while others discover this path through a dream or vision. Selection is based on signs of devotion, wisdom, humility, and honesty. Once called, the individual seeks training, usually by apprenticing to a medicine person for a number of years. All knowledge comes from the Creator, and the elders are charged with the responsibility of keeping knowledge about healing foods, herbs, and medicine and passing it on. Trusted with all secrets, rituals, and legends of their people, Native healers are considered to be inspired individuals with great importance to the tribe. Training is complete when the teacher says it is complete and when the candidate has practiced the skills publicly and with success.

Medicine people believe that the healing knowledge they possess has to be dispensed in a certain way, often through ritual or ceremony. Healers receive their knowledge through fasting and asking for guidance from Above. During the period of fasting, the Great Being might reveal a chant or the location of a particular herb and give instructions on how to use it for different illnesses.

Time is often considered an ally in recovery. With the passage of time, fears and problems sometimes fade. Love is a key element in the healing process. The healer enters into the healing relationship with love and compassion. The two individuals experience a joining or merging as this process unfolds. This merger symbolizes the cementing together of people and the Divine Spirit.

The Circle

The circle represents the cycles of life that have no beginning, no end, and no time element. The Great Spirit causes everything to be round. The sun, earth, and moon are round. The sky is deep like a bowl. Things that grow from the ground like the stem of a plant or plant roots are round. The circle, symbol of infinity and interconnectedness, is seen in the sweatlodge, the bowl of the Sacred Pipe, the Sacred Hoop, and the Medicine Wheel. In addition, the camp is circular, tepees are circular, and people sit in a circle in all ceremonies. When people come together in a circle, a spirit of oneness and a sense of sacredness come upon them.

The Medicine Wheel is both an important conceptual scheme and a major ceremonial observance. The Sacred Hoop makes up the circumference with the interior of the circle being divided into four quadrants. Each quadrant represents a direction, a totem, an element, a color, a kingdom, a quality, a season, and a gateway to the individual. The four colors—white, black, yellow, and red—represent the races of all humanity. See Figure 5.1 for an illustration of the Medicine Wheel.

FIGURE 5.1

The Medicine Wheel: center of Native American healing.

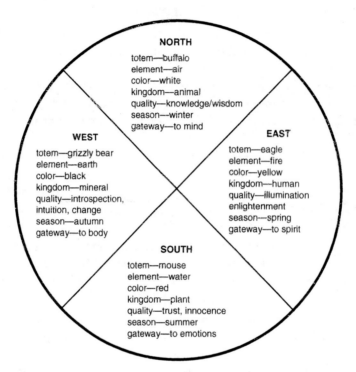

NORTH
totem—buffalo
element—air
color—white
kingdom—animal
quality—knowledge/wisdom
season—winter
gateway—to mind

WEST
totem—grizzly bear
element—earth
color—black
kingdom—mineral
quality—introspection,
intuition, change
season—autumn
gateway—to body

EAST
totem—eagle
element—fire
color—yellow
kingdom—human
quality—illumination
enlightenment
season—spring
gateway—to spirit

SOUTH
totem—mouse
element—water
color—red
kingdom—plant
quality—trust, innocence
season—summer
gateway—to emotions

The Number Four

The number four is significant to Native American people and is incorporated into their daily lives through prayers, ceremonies, and activities. It is believed to be the number of completeness. Everything that grows from the earth consists of four parts: roots, stems, leaves, and fruit. Earth, air, fire, and water are the four elements. Four types of things take breath: those that crawl, those that fly, those that walk on four legs, and those that walk on two legs. There are four directions, four seasons, and four races of people—white, black, yellow, and red.

Harmony with All Things: The Native American View of Health and Illness

Health is viewed as a balance or harmony of mind and body. The goal is to be in harmony with all things, which means first being in harmony with oneself. Harmony is thought to neutralize problems and help one's life to become beautiful. Good health makes it easier for all people to do their part in the universe, to serve others, and to fulfill their personal life visions.

Life is considered in all of its dualities: winter/summer, cold/hot, day/night, mind/body, spiritual/physical, work/play, and so on. Native people believe that the two sides of everything deserve equal attention and that both should be nourished with love. A healthy person who is walking in balance is energized and alert, and even in the presence of disease will still feel alive and fulfilled.

Traditionally, Native American people lived long, happy, healthy, and balanced lives. They did everything to respect and honor Mother Earth and the Great Spirit. They ate wholesome food and considered all food to be blessed as a gift of life from the Creator. They got up with the sun and went to bed with the moon. Exercise was a natural part of their lives, integrated into daily activities. These good health habits, a sense of joy, and a purpose in life are key factors for living into old age.

Illness occurs when balance is disrupted. It is believed that most illness begins in the head and that people must get rid of ideas that predispose illness. If the mind is negative, the body will be drained, making it more vulnerable. When people open up to the universe, learn what is good for them, and find ways to be happier, they can begin to work toward a longer and healthier life. Many ancient people had ways to get rid of this negativity. The Mayan people of Mexico would stand in a stream of flowing water and talk out all their angers, fears, sorrows, or troubles over the water. The moving water would take all the emotions they poured out of themselves into the current and away from them.

Role of Medicine Women and Men

Although they are the primary care providers in many places, the responsibilities of medicine women and men go beyond healing illness. They also evaluate advice and treatment given by other health care practitioners. They often have a strong influence on the acceptance or rejection of the treatment plans from conventional health care providers. They may also function as tribal social mediators, dispensing traditional wisdom and suggesting action. Medicine people reaffirm and strengthen tribal identity through the recounting of myth and song. They have an extensive knowledge of their communities and of family relationships and interaction. They are the formulators and teachers of the old religion and creators of the new. Medicine people are figures of authority and awe as instruments of the Creator.

How Does Native American Medicine Work?

Native American healers place a premium on identifying the true source of the problem, so they can treat the cause, not just the effect. They always look at the total person, whether they are treating someone for physical illness or emotional problems. They look at the overall picture, determine what is out of balance within the whole, and then pinpoint the trouble spots. Some healers diagnose by going into trance. While in trance, "hand tremblers" pass their shaking hands over the body of the person; when the hands stop trembling, the locale of the illness is found and the cause is usually identified. "Star gazers" also enter trance states to read cause in the stars. "Listeners" do not go into trance but listen to the person's story and on that basis identify the cause of the illness.

When people fall ill, they often experience anxiety and fear that may incapacitate them. The healer is not so burdened and is able to supply coherence, calmness, and hope. Power flows through the healer to the patient. Healers use medicine objects to assist them, and treatments consist of ceremony, touch, herbs, and sometimes peyote.

Items used to help make medicine are called *medicine objects*. Medicine objects can be anything that relates to the Great Spirit in a sacred way. The medicine bag contains healing objects, which vary in size and number but typically contain such things as feathers, claws, bird or animal bones, an assortment of herbs or roots, smudges, or paints. The medicine bag may also contain personal items that represent one's self and personal experiences and are sacred to the individual. Native Americans believe that their medicine bags carry a part of themselves and are among their most prized companions. The Medicine Wheel is a sacred circle usually built from stones. It is entered for the purpose of healing, giving thanks, praying, or meditating. The Pipe is one of the most sacred medicine objects and is an instrument of prayer.

The Native American art of healing is ceremonial in nature. Different ceremonies are conducted according to the type of illness or the severity of the person's condition. Medicine people or holy people lead the healing ceremonies. The primary purpose is to allow connection with the Great Healer, since physical health often fails without the aid of spiritual means. A secondary benefit is a cleansing of the body, mind, and spirit. A healing session is never a casual encounter. It is arranged through a formalized procedure after discussion by the patient, family, advisors, and healer. Acceptance by the healer is followed by instructions on preliminary actions that may include fasting, abstinences, prayers, or the preparation of offerings or feasts. Some more specific healing practices are described below.

Smudging

Smudging is a cleansing and purifying process using smoke from burning herbs, usually sweet grass, sage, or cedar. People and all sacred objects are smudged so all can be centered and focused on the healing process. The smoke clears negativity, purifies the energy field of people and places, and is a prayer to the Creator. In addition to use in healing ceremonies, smudging is used in the morning or evening as part of daily devotion. Smudging is a practice known to many religions; examples include the use of frankincense in Catholic churches and sticks of incense in Buddhist temples.

Sweatlodge

The sweatlodge is a ceremony to cleanse body, mind, heart, and spirit. It may be held on its own or in preparation for another ceremony, such as a vision quest. Typically, the sweatlodge is held in a round structure covered with overlapped pieces of tarpaulin or blankets with a small door flap. When the flap is down, the place is nearly dark and almost sealed off from the outer air. Near the lodge is a fire pit, where rocks are heated and then passed into the lodge. Water from a bucket is splashed on the stones, creating a dense steam referred to as the Breath of Spirit. Depending on the illness, a variety of herbs are burned on the sweat rocks. Sacred songs and prayers go on for several hours. Everyone in the sweatlodge prays hard for the one needing healing, but it is the responsibility of the one being healed to pray that healing energies come to her/him and ask the Spirit to give guidance to the medicine person.

The sweatlodge is also a powerful ceremony for keeping people healthy, and many view it as the first line of defense in preventing illness. It is a bringing together of the four elements: earth, air, fire, and water. Through sweating and praying, the body is cleansed of toxins, the mind of negativities, the heart of hatred, and the spirit of doubt. The sweatlodge is as a sacred a place as a church or temple.

Drumming and Chanting

Drumming and chanting are powerful ways to bring oneself in balance with self, others, and the world. Drumming harmonizes people with the heartbeat of Mother Earth. It is a pulse rather than a tempo. As people dance to the pulse of the drum, they dance in harmony with the Creator and with one another. Symbolically, the drum represents all life. The wood was once a tree, and the skin covering the drum was once life. They are related to life that has gone on, yet they are helping the lives that are still here. Chanting is a form of prayer through music. Holyway chants are used to attract good, to cure, and to repair; ghostway chants are used to remove evil; lifeway chants are used to treat injuries and accidents.

Sing

A sing is a healing ceremony that lasts from two to nine days and nights. A highly skilled specialist called a singer guides the ceremony. Used in healing, sings are attended by as many people in the community as possible because just being present is considered healing. Some songs are only for children and call on spirits who take care of little children. Some spiritual songs take care of adults only. Other songs focus on specific problems, such as the song for small burns that will cool them and keep them from blistering. To learn a single chant can take up to several years. It takes some people 40 years of singing before they master the chants and the accompanying herbal preparations.

Pipe Ceremony

The Pipe ceremony takes many different forms depending on how this sacred knowledge was given to the various tribes. The Pipe is one of the most sacred medicine objects and represents the universe to Native American people. The bowl represents Earth Mother and the female powers of the universe. The stem represents the plant kingdom and the male powers of the universe. When the bowl and stem are joined together, the Pipe is sacred. The tobacco smoked in the Pipe is an instrument of prayer and has come to signify the sacredness of the ritual. As the smoke of the Pipe rises, it creates an atmosphere of prayer by symbolizing prayers going up to the Creator.

Pipes are used for private and group prayers. Prayers are transmitted in the smoke of the burning tobacco. Participants in the Pipe ceremony are as centered and focused as possible, since everything they think and feel is part of the prayers being offered. As in many other ceremonies, the number four has special significance. The Pipe is offered to the four directions and is often passed in four ritual repetitions.

Vision Quest

An extremely powerful ceremony is the Vision Quest. Traditionally, it is a time of fasting, praying, isolation, and exposure to the elements, all of which contribute to a mystic experience with the goal of understanding self and communicating with the Great Spirit. Questions are asked, such as How can I best serve the people? How can I best serve Mother Earth? How can I best serve future generations? The Vision Quest tells people who they are, what they are really supposed to do, what their life goal should be, and the purpose and meaning of their lives. The Vision Quest begins with a sweatlodge for purification, after which the person is taken to an isolated place in nature and begins the period of silence and fasting. During the Vision Quest, the individual focuses only on prayer and vision and in this way is pushed into the spirit world. After the Vision Quest, the person returns to the sweatlodge and a Pipe Ceremony.

Healing Touch/Acupressure

Native Americans have always considered touch to be therapeutic. The Creator touches patients and transfers power to them through medicine people or shamans who are healing instruments. Touching, an expression of loving care, is essential for the healing process. It cleanses the affected area and relieves pain. The healer's willingness to touch demonstrates no fear of contamination. Healing touch is a powerful way to remove barriers and create or restore relationships.

Some tribes have used a form of acupressure since ancient times. Compared with traditional Chinese practitioners, Native Americans use fewer pressure points but a similar process. Prior to using acupressure, medicine people warm their hands over a fire so that the Great Being can send healing warmth through them to the patient. It is believed that no harm will be done to a person as long as the pressure is applied slowly and in a relaxed way. Medicine people are taught that acupressure should only be done with the utmost gentleness and love.

Herbs

Native Americans have long used herbs in maintaining health and treating disease. Botanical remedies are supplemented with ceremony and prayer during the healing process. The beneficial properties of herbs as medicines often depend on the greenness or ripeness of the plant and the part of the plant to be used such as roots, barks, twigs, bulbs, rhizomes, fruit seed, tubers, leaves, and flowers. Knowing the best time for cutting and digging each type of plant, for peak effectiveness, is part of the knowledge of the Native healer. Whether it be in summer, winter, spring, or autumn, the timing must be appropriate for each plant. An herb gathered with prayers, at the correct time and prepared properly will restore a person from illness to health.

Ancient Native people considered nature to be their pharmacy. They did not have aspirin but they did have willow bark, which contains salicylic acid. The active ingredient in squaw tea is ephedrine, the main ingredient in many cold cures now on the conventional market. The active ingredient in foxglove is digitalis, which was used to brew tea to help people with heart problems. Particular molds, similar to those forming the basis for penicillin, were used to treat infections. Purple coneflower (echinacea) is an immune system booster and antibiotic, which is held in high esteem by many people today. Goldenseal, which is a good disinfectant that promotes scab formation, is one of the most important Native American medicinal plants. Currently, it is also used as a gargle for sore throat or as a mouth rinse for canker sores, tonsillitis, and infected gums. More information about herbal cures can be found in Chapter 6, "Herbal Medicine."

Peyote

The hallucinogenic herb, peyote, has been used by the Native Americans of North America for a long time. Native people do not use peyote to "get high" but rather to see teaching visions. Peyote makes people highly sensitive to sight and sound and more aware of what is around and inside of them. It is used to heal all kinds of sickness, for clairvoyance, and in the worship of the Great Being. It is believed that the Creator put peyote on earth as a medicine to help people. It is viewed somewhat like an aspirin, a cure for all kinds of physical as well as mental and emotional problems.

How Can I Get Started with Native American Healing?

Although the modern Native American population might not initially seem to be an exemplar of good health practices, it's important to separate the tradition and potential of Native American culture with its current situation. Adopting the traditions of gratitude and reverence for nature is a great way to begin adopting a Native American attitude toward one's health. Several mental exercises to cultivate these attitudes are presented below, and the resources section lists avenues for further exploration.

Fostering Positive Thoughts

Just as Native American tribes have rituals for cleansing the mind of negative thoughts and feelings, which predispose to disease, we can develop our own rituals to modify unhealthy thinking patterns. Negative thinking not only occurs in our brains, but it also occurs in our bodies; negative thoughts cause instantaneous chemical changes in every cell. Continuous cellular disruption may contribute to the onset of illness and disease. To counteract negative thinking, you may find it helpful to look at yourself in the mirror and say aloud, three good things about yourself. People might say, "I'm a good friend," "I'm an honest person," "I'm a caring person," "My hair looks beautiful today," "I am becoming healthier every day," and so on. The goal is to say different positive qualities about themselves each day. Keeping a journal about feelings immediately after the exercise and feelings throughout the day is helpful in evaluating the impact of positive statements on negative thinking.

Positive affirmations are another way to counteract negative thinking. Make a list of positive things in your life, including things you would like to occur. Affirmations are always stated as if they were a fact, even when they are still a dream. For example, if you have financial problems, instead of thinking "I'm never going to get ahead. My debts are just too big," you might make affirmations such as "I am financially secure," "I pay my bills easily," "Money comes in when I need it," "I am at ease about the subject of money." Affirmations can be made about work, school, relationships, feelings, commitments, future goals, and even pleasurable activities. Write your list of affirmations over a period of several days, then find a time and place to say them aloud every day. You may want to tape record them and listen to the tape every day, perhaps to make a commute to work more pleasant. Since people tend to live their lives according to their expectations, changing expectations from negative to positive can improve the level of wellness.

Banishing Negative Thoughts

Often we endure such runs of negative thoughts that we are unaware of the process until we have been "beating ourselves up" for 10–15 minutes. To become more aware of this habitual process, tap your left finger on a firm surface for every negative thought. When your finger becomes quite sore, you will have another level of awareness of your negativity. Negative thoughts can be countered with positive ones. When you catch yourself thinking and feeling a negative thought, such as how fat your body is or how dumb you are, STOP. Now look for and substitute a positive thought or feeling in the place of the one you removed, such as how lovely your hair looks or how well you have succeeded at something. Now listen to yourself saying the positive phrase out loud. Continue in this way, adding other phrases and wishes.

Although it might not be easy to find a stream of flowing water to take away your angers, fears, sorrows, or troubles, you can visualize that process. Relax yourself with deep breathing and by banishing negative thoughts, then mentally walk into a stream or actually stand in a shower that is comfortable in temperature and flow. Visualize the water washing out all their physical, mental, emotional, or relational problems. Feel a Native-American-style gratitude toward nature and creation, and feel grateful to yourself, for spending time and energy on this ritual healing.

THE ABSOLUTE MINIMUM

- Native American medicine creates healing experiences by deepening the connection and understanding between the patient and the natural world.

- Ritual has a vital place in Native American healing, with ceremonies such as the sweatlodge, pipe ceremony, and vision quest being used by medicine men and women to increase the natural balance that leads to healing.

- Although poor health is now chronic in much of the Native American community, increased interest by the alternative medical community and consumers is creating a renaissance in Native American healing.

RESOURCES

- Bear Heart, *The Wind Is My Mother*, Berkley Books, New York, 1996

- Dance of the Deer Foundation

  www.shamanism.com

- The School of Lost Borders (Vision Quests)

  www.schooloflostborders.com

- The Featured Pipe Ranch

  www.featheredpipe.com/ranch

PART III

BOTANICAL HEALING

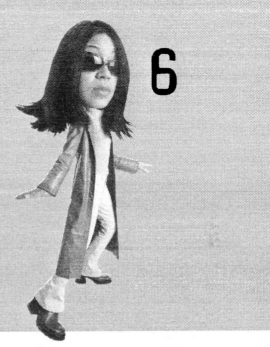

6

HERBAL MEDICINE

Also known as botanical medicine or *phytotherapy* (phyto means plant), herbal medicine is used by 80 percent of the world's population. According to a national survey by *Prevention* magazine, adults in the United States spend an average of $54 a year on herbs, resulting in a $3.24 billion-a-year business. In some cases, herbal alternatives are giving prescription drugs a run for their money. For many conditions, herbs are the treatment of choice because they are milder and have fewer side effects than prescription drugs. In the past, herbal medicines were available only in health food stores, but they now can be found in mainstream supermarkets and pharmacies.

What Is Herbal Medicine?

Throughout history, almost all societies have used plants for therapeutic purposes. For example, the oldest surviving prescription, carved into a clay tablet and dating from 3000 BC, is for garlic. Over thousands of years, a medical pharmacopoeia developed in every culture, from Asia to the Americas, to Europe and Africa. Over an extensive period of time, Chinese herbalists documented the healing properties of more than 7,000 herbs and thousands of herbal combinations. St. John's wort has a 2,500-year history of safe and effective use and was prescribed as medicine by Hippocrates (460–377 BC) himself, though, of course, he had a different name for it. Galen (130–200 AD) described 130 herbal antidotes and medicines, and Dioscorides (first century AD) wrote about the medicinal properties of 500 plants and described how to prepare 1,000 simple remedies. The ancient Egyptians used peppermint and spearmint to relax the digestive tract, while Chinese and Ayurvedic doctors used mint to treat colds, coughs, and fevers.

When Europeans came to the Americas, they found that Native Americans had a vast pharmacopeia of medicinal plants such as birch, blackberry, coneflower, ginseng, goldenseal, and ginger, handed down from generation to generation. Early Jesuit missionaries in Canada discovered American ginseng in the early 1700s and exported it to Asia where it became a highly revered tonic. The Shakers (Church of the United Society of Believers), who were great friends of Native Americans, were the first to cultivate medicinal plants in mass quantities and became the first reputable pharmaceutical manufacturers in the United States. Until the Civil War disrupted their efforts, they were selling 354 varieties of therapeutic herbs.

During the early 20th century, tincture of echinacea was highly valued for its antibiotic properties until synthetic antibiotics became available. Kava, used to calm the nervous system and decrease anxiety, was even sold in the Sears, Roebuck and Co. catalog during the 1920s. Many herbs used in ancient times are still in use today throughout the world. Herbal medicine has generally been more widely accepted outside the United States, where health care providers often combine it with conventional therapy.

Researchers are intensifying their efforts to collect and screen more natural products for their medicinal properties. Gordon Cragg, chief of the National Cancer Institute's natural-products branch states, "Nature produces chemicals that no chemist would ever dream of at the laboratory bench." The most concentrated and diverse number of healing herbs is found in a wide band around the equator. Unfortunately, destruction of these natural plant habitats, especially tropical rain forests, is driving many species to extinction before they can be found and studied.

Much of what is known about herbs comes from Germany, where an expert panel called Commission E, set up in 1978, reviewed all available literature on 300 medicinal herbs, issuing recommendations for their use. Several smaller pharmaceutical companies in the United States, such as Shaman Pharmaceuticals, are working closely with native herbalists in a number of countries. In addition, the National

Cancer Institute (NCI) is screening plants for compounds active against the AIDS virus and nine major types of cancer. Since 1986, the NCI has received samplings of thousands of plants from ethnobotanists throughout the world. Indigenous people have been testing and using healing plants for thousands of years but only recently have their knowledge been sought by Western researchers.

REGULATING HERBAL MEDICINE IN THE UNITED STATES

In the 1960s, the Food and Drug Administration (FDA) developed the current U.S. regulations regarding medications. At that time, herbal medicine had little popularity and thus was virtually ignored by the FDA. Herbs are viewed as dietary supplements and are controlled by the 1994 Dietary Supplement Health and Education Act. Under this act, dietary supplements cannot make specific medical claims as can prescription and OTC drugs. General statements such as "improves memory" or "promotes regularity" can be used as long as a disclaimer notes that the herb is not approved by the FDA and that the product is not intended to diagnose, treat, cure, or prevent any disease.

It is unlikely that most herbal medicines will ever win FDA approval since the process costs approximately $100 million per drug. Large pharmaceutical companies are willing to invest this fortune in new drugs that can be patented and sold at high profits. In contrast, granting exclusive rights or patents to most herbs, such as garlic or ginseng, is nearly impossible, which takes away the financial incentive to get them approved for medicinal use. The lack of profit, rather than the lack of efficacy of herbs, keeps drug companies from advocating change toward FDA approval of herbs.

How Does Herbal Medicine Work?

Herbal medicine is the original medicine. In many parts of the world, treating illness with herbs is still the only medicine available. Even though only a tiny fraction of plants have been studied for medicinal benefits, conventional physicians regularly use plant-derived products. Twenty-five percent of all prescription drugs sold in the United States are derived from plants. Examples of herbal remedies that have been synthesized into modern drugs are reserpine from Indian snakeroot, digoxin from foxglove, quinine from Peruvian bark, aspirin from willow tree bark, morphine from opium poppy, cocaine from coca leaves, and atropine from deadly nightshade. Recently, researchers discovered taxol, found in Pacific yew bark, which is currently being used in the treatment of early and advanced breast cancer and ovarian tumors. Taxol has also been found to decrease the chances of developing breast cancer in women who are at high risk. Unfortunately, taxol has also been associated with an increased risk for pulmonary embolism and endometrial cancer. Another recent advance is the drug vincristine, which has been isolated from the Madagascar periwinkle. Vincristine has been found to arrest cell division so dramatically that it is being used to treat acute leukemia and Hodgkin's disease.

Phytonutrients

Phytonutrients are chemicals present in plants that make the plants biologically active and are responsible for giving plants their color, flavor, and natural disease resistance. Phytonutrients are products of photosynthesis or are substances that serve as defense mechanisms against attacks by insects and other predators. These active components of plants usually occur in groups that complement the protective and healing effects of each other. Descriptions of the most important phytonutrients and their uses are found in Table 6.1.

Table 6.1 Phytonutrients

Phytonutrient	Properties	Use & Effects
Carbohydrates	Main energy source and structural support of plants	In some herbs, such as coltsfood and marshmallow, the cellulose combines with other chemicals to form mucilage, a gummy substance, which, when ingested by humans, soothes and protects irritated or inflamed internal tissue.
Fatty oils	Mixture of triglycerides, glycerol, and fatty acids	Cathartic effect of castor oil useful for constipation and colic in young children.
Essential oils	Vaporize when heated; combinations give plants their particular smell	Garlic is an antiseptic, thyme is an expectorant, chamomile relieves gaseous distention and painful intestinal spasms.
Tannins	Chemical substances with astringent and antiseptic properties	Form a protective layer on the skin and mucous membranes and are useful in treatment of burns and local inflammation; used for eye and mouth infections.
Bitter principles	Group of chemicals that have an extremely bitter taste	Through a reflex action via tastebuds, stimulate appetite and flow of digestive juices, stimulate liver activity and flow of bile, some act as diuretics. Viewed as overall tonics.

Phytonutrient	Properties	Use & Effects
Alkaloids	Group of nitrogen-containing compounds with most therapeutic plant substances: analgesic, local anesthetic, sedating, antispasmodic, heart constricting, and/or hallucinatory; poisonous to varying degrees	Affect both the nervous and circulatory systems. Most familiar are atropine, caffeine, cocaine, morphine, nicotine, and quinine.
Isoflavones	Compounds similar to human estrogen and found primarily in soy products	May prevent prostate, breast, and other hormone-related cancers; lower cholesterol, relieve menopausal symptoms, prevent osteoporosis by increasing bone density.
Carotenoids	Yellow, orange, or red pigments in photosynthetic plants, converted into vitamin A in the liver	Beta-carotene may aid in cancer prevention by neutralizing free radicals. Used in conjunction with topical sunscreens, better prevention of sunburn and skin damage.
		Lycopene may prevent prostate cancer and decrease risk of heart attacks.
		Lutein may be useful in prevention of macular degeneration, a leading cause of blindness in the elderly.
Glycosides	Complex organic substances; some of most potent herbal remedies and among most toxic substance known	Cardiac glycosides include foxglove and lily of the valley, which affect cardiac contractions and used to correct arrhythmias.
		Mustard glycosides are used externally and have antiseptic and analgesic effects.
		Cyanogenic glycosides release hydrogen cyanide when chewed or digested resulting in antispasmodic, purgative, and sedative effects. Found in some nuts, vegetables, and the seeds of some fruits. Hydrogen cyanide, sometimes called prussic acid, is highly poisonous.
		Phenolic glycosides include salicylic derivatives found in willow and other plants and is main ingredient in aspirin–antiseptic, analgesic, and anti-inflammatory effects.
		Coumarine glycosides strengthen capillary walls and act as anticoagulant.
		Anthraquinones glycosides are used as laxatives.

Antioxidants

Antioxidants are a group of vitamins, minerals, enzymes, and herbs that help protect the body from naturally occurring free radicals. As the body goes through its normal processes, in which oxygen is used to provide cellular fuel, some of the oxygen molecules lose one of their electrons. When they do, the formerly stable oxygen molecules become dangerous free radicals that then try to stabilize themselves by stealing another electron from stable molecules, thus damaging them and creating more free radicals. Because free radicals react so easily with other compounds, they can effect significant changes in the body. Many different factors can lead to the production of free radicals. Internal sources, in addition to oxygen consumption, include emotional stress and strenuous exercise. External sources include air pollution, cigarette smoke, factory and car exhaust, smog, pesticides, herbicides, food contaminants, chemotherapy, and radiation. All cause the overproduction of free radicals.

Oxidative damage can be visualized by biting into an apple. After a few minutes, the exposed part becomes brown, and that's oxidization in action. Unfortunately, we cannot "see" the damage being done by free radicals in our bodies. An excess of free radicals is, in part, responsible for the effects of aging and is implicated in cancer and a variety of chronic and degenerative conditions, including arthritis and heart disease.

Free radicals are normally kept under control through the production of enzymes that act as free radical scavengers, searching out and neutralizing dangerous free radicals. As people age, they produce fewer of these enzymes, and may benefit from dietary antioxidants such as vitamin C, vitamin E, carotenoids, the mineral selenium, and the hormone melatonin. Herbs with antioxidant properties include bilberry, ginkgo, grape seed extract, green tea, and flavonoids. Fruits and vegetables are the primary sources for antioxidants, though they are also available in the form of supplements.

Synergism

The active chemicals in herbs work synergistically–that is, the action of two or more substances achieves an effect of which they are incapable individually. Most herbal medicines rely on the complex interplay of many chemicals for the therapeutic action and many lose their activity when purified and isolated. For example, a number of antimicrobial compounds are found in tea tree oil, but studies indicate that no single compound in the oil accomplishes its remarkable germ-fighting ability; rather, the interaction of at least eight distinct chemicals in the oil seems to produce the effects.

This complexity makes it nearly impossible for an infectious microbe to build up resistance to tea tree oil. One of the primary problems with conventional antibiotics is the ability of many microbes to develop resistance, thus rendering the drug useless.

Antioxidant defenses also operate synergistically. For example, a number of carotenoids working together have higher anticancer properties than a single carotenoid. Thus beta-carotene supplements may not provide the same protection as eating fruits and vegetables rich in beta-carotene. Other substances in the plant may help the body to assimilate its benefits as well as buffer any side effects. Including the whole plant in the final product often ensures that some measure of the natural "checks and balances" will be retained.

Various herbs and other substances may also work synergistically with one another. A rather dramatic example of this effect occurred during the testing of plant samples from the rain forest of Ecuador for chemicals that could be used to treat diabetes. The leaves from the plant were immersed in an alcohol extract and then a water extract. The debate among the researchers concerned whether to throw a live crab into the extract, just as native healers did. Some believed it might make a difference while others believed the crab was simply ritualistic. Amazingly, the only extract that showed therapeutic effect was the one with the crab in it. It turns out that a component in a crab's shell is needed to extract the active chemical compound from the plant.

Safety

Not all plant life is beneficial. Most plant-related poisonings are due to accidental consumption of toxic ornamental plants such as jade, holly, poinsettia, schefflera, philodendron, and dieffenbachia rather than from herbs. Data compiled by the American Association of Poison Control Centers indicates that in any two-year period of time, plants cause two or three deaths and approximately 50 major poisonings. In contrast, prescription medications cause close to a thousand deaths from poisoning and almost 7,000 major nonfatal poisonings per year. Unrelated to direct poisoning are adverse drug reactions (ADRs), defined as any unintended and undesired effect of a drug with usual therapeutic doses. After excluding errors in drug administration, noncompliance, overdose, and drug abuse, a significant study found that ADRs may be the fourth to sixth leading cause of death in the United States. This incidence has remained stable over the past 30 years, a fact not widely recognized by the general population.

The vast majority of herbal medicines present no danger. Some can, however, cause serious side effects if taken in excess or, for some, if taken over a prolonged period of time. For example, comfrey, a digestive remedy, and coltsfoot, used to treat cough, can cause liver damage if taken in large doses. Herbs can also interact with drugs, and caution should be used when combining herbs with prescription and OTC medications. With the exception of mild herb teas, pregnant women should not take herbs internally.

How Can I Get Started with Herbal Medicine?

Medicinal herbs are available at health food stores, herb shops, supermarkets, and pharmacies. They can be used as a preventative, a tonic, or a treatment. Herbs can be prepared and used in a number of ways. *Extracts* or *tinctures* are made by pressing herbs with a heavy press and soaking them in alcohol or water, which after evaporation yields a concentrated extract. Extracts are generally measured in drops and diluted in a small amount of water for ingestion. A preparation of the delicate parts of plants—that is, leaves, flowers, and seeds—is called an *infusion*, a process similar to making tea. Hot water is poured over the herb, steeped for 3–5 minutes, and strained before drinking. Honey or lemon may be added to taste. *Decoction* is the preparation of the more resilient parts of plants, such as the bark, roots, and berries. These parts of the herb are usually boiled for 10–20 minutes and strained before drinking. A *compress* is a cloth soaked in a warm or cool herbal solution and applied directly to an injured area. An herbal *poultice* is made by mixing powered herbs with enough hot water to make a thick paste that is then applied directly to the skin. Poultices are used to reduce swelling, relieve pain, decrease muscle spasms, draw out toxins from the body, increase circulation, and speed healing. Table 6.2 lists some of the more common herbs as well as their action, dosage, and side effects. Table 6.3 provides some herbal remedies you can make at home.

Table 6.2 Common Herbal Treatments

Herb	Properties/Use	Form/Dose	Notes
Capsaicin	For tenderness and pain of osteoarthritis, fibromyalgia, diabetic neuropathy, shingles	Cream topically applied	May be a brief burning or stinging sensation with first use; wash hands after applying; avoid touching eyes
Chamomile	For anxiety, stomach distress, stomach ulcers, infant colic, drug withdrawal	Infusion or tincture, 1 teaspoon twice daily	NOT for those allergic to ragweed
Chondroitin	Helps slow cartilage degradation in osteoarthritis	400 mg twice daily	No known side effects
Echinacea	Antiviral, antibiotic for colds, flu, and other infections	400 mg for 5–14 days, peaks at 5 days	NOT for people with autoimmune disease; NOT for pregnant and lactating women; bitter taste

Herb	Properties/Use	Form/Dose	Notes
Evening Primrose oil	For PMS, mastalgia, hypertension, multiple sclerosis, alcoholism	250–500 mg/day	No known side effects
Feverfew	For prevention of migraines	0.2% parthenolide, 100–300 mg/day	NOT for use with prescription headache drugs; NOT for use by pregnant and lactating women; as chewing leaves can cause mouth sores and loss of taste, capsule forms are preferred
Garlic	Antibiotic, antiviral, antifungal, anticoagulant; for any infection, hypertension, high blood lipid levels	Varying recommendations	NOT for people with blood clotting disorders; may cause stomach upset
Ginger	For nausea and vomiting of various causes, hypertension, high cholesterol; enhances insulin	500–1000 mg every 4 hrs (for motion sickness, take 1500 mg 30 minutes before travel)	People taking anticoagulant should check with MD prior to use
Ginkgo	For attention and memory problems, headaches, tinnitus, intermittent claudication, erectile problems	24% flavonoids & 6% terpenes, 60—80 mg three or four times daily	May cause mild GI upset
Ginseng	For mood swings, improved physical performance, reduction of fasting blood glucose, stimulation of immune system, ease cocaine withdrawal	200 mg twice daily, for at least 4–6 weeks	NOT for use when acutely ill with cold or flu; NOT to be used with hypoglycemia; may cause nervousness, insomnia, euphoria, or hypertension
Glucosamine	Improves pain and movement in osteoarthritis	500 mg three times daily	People taking diuretics may need higher doses of herb
Goldenseal	Antibiotic, antiseptic, anti-inflammatory for wound healing, colds and flu, hypertension, uterine bleeding, enhances insulin	2 capsules three times daily, for no more than 3 weeks	NOT for use during pregnancy–may cause premature uterine contractions; only for short-term use; long-term use may irritate or inflame mucosa

Table 6.2   Continued

Herb	Properties/Use	Form/Dose	Notes
Green tea	Antioxidant, protects against cancer, lowers cholesterol, helps regulate blood sugar and insulin levels	3–4 cups/day	NOT to be used in large quantities during pregnancy, people with anxiety disorder or irregular heartbeat should limit use to no more than 2 cups daily
Kava	For anxiety, insomnia, low energy, muscle tension	100 mg three times daily	Intoxicating in large amounts, with potential for abuse
Milk Thistle	Antioxidant for all liver disorders; psoriasis	Varying	No known side effects
St. John's Wort	For mild to moderate depression, viral infections including HIV and herpes	900 mg/day, for at least 4–8 weeks	NOT for pregnant and lactating women, not for children; NOT for use with other antidepressants; may cause photosensitivity; avoid foods with tyramine and OTC cold and flu remedies, amino acid supplements
Saw Palmetto	Urinary antiseptic, for benign prostatic hyperplasia	160 mg twice daily	Use only after proper diagnosis from primary practitioner; may cause dizziness, dry mouth, tachycardia, angina, testicular pain
Selenium	Antioxidant especially when combined with vitamin E, may prevent some types of tumors, aids in production of antibodies, protects liver	200 mcg	Excessively high levels may lead to liver and kidney impairment; causes metallic taste in mouth, garlicky breath odor
Tea Tree Oil	Antifungal, antiseptic, for acne, minor burns and cuts, athlete's foot, nail infections, herpes, douche for yeast infections	Full strength or dilute in water or oil	For external use; do NOT ingest

Herb	Properties/Use	Form/Dose	Notes
Valerian	For insomnia, muscle pain, menstrual and intestinal cramps, benzodiazepine withdrawal	400 mg before bed 0.5% essential oil	NOT to be used with alcohol, nonaddictive; bitter taste
Yohimbe	For decreased sex drive, erectile problems	Varying	NOT for people with hypertension, kidney disease; NOT to be used with tyramines, OTC cold remedies, caffeine; may cause hypertension, anxiety, panic attacks, hallucinations

Table 6.3   Herbal Remedies to Make at Home

Herb	Uses	Preparations
Borage	Used for reducing fever and also for increasing milk in nursing mothers.	Combine a small handful of fresh leaves with 2 1/2 cups boiling water. Steep 10 minutes, strain, and drink warm.
Chamomile	An excellent home remedy for indigestion, heartburn, and infant colic. It also soothes skin and has mild relaxant and sedative properties.	For an infusion, use 2–3 heaping teaspoons of dried or 1/3 cup of fresh flowers per cup of boiling water. Steep 10–20 minutes. Strain and drink up to 3 cups a day. Diluted infusions may be given to infants for colic.
		For a relaxing herbal bath, fill a cloth bag with a few handfuls of dried or fresh flowers and let the water run over it.
		For allergic skin rashes, tightly pack a jar of flower heads, cover with olive oil, cover, and set in a sunny place for 3 weeks. Strain and apply to rashes.
Comfrey	External use only. Promotes the growth of new cells and has a mild anti-inflammatory action. Used in wound and burn treatment.	Mix powdered root with water to make a paste. Apply to injured area and cover with clean bandage. Change daily.

Table 6.3   Continued

Herb	Uses	Preparations
Ginger	Decreases nausea, boosts the immune system, lowers blood pressure.	Use 2 teaspoons of powdered or grated root per cup of boiling water. Steep 20 minutes, strain; add juice from half a lemon and honey to taste. Drink hot up to 3 cups a day. Dilute ginger infusion to treat infant colic. If you buy whole root, refrigerate it.
Mint	Relaxes the digestive tract; used to treat colds, coughs, and fevers.	For an infusion, use 1 teaspoon of fresh herb or 2 teaspoons of dried leaves per cup of boiling water. Steep 10 minutes, strain, and drink up to 3 cups a day. Peppermint has a sharper taste than spearmint and feels cooler in the mouth. For a relaxing herbal bath, fill a cloth bag with a few handfuls of dried or fresh leaves and let the water run over it.
Rosemary	Stimulates circulation and relaxes tired and sore muscles.	For tired, sore feet, make a footbath by adding 10 drops of essential oil to a basin of hot water large enough to hold both feet. Stir the oil into the water with your hand

Putting Herbs in Perspective

Because herbs are marketed as "natural" or promoted as foods, consumers may assume incorrectly that herbs are safe and without side effects. It is important that you remember that natural remedies should be approached with respect. They work because they have strong pharmacological activity. And while herbs are generally much safer than prescription drugs, if you abuse or overuse them, they can cause harm.

Although herbs can be quite effective, it is also important to not become fanatical. If you have a life-threatening illness such as asthma, experience chest pain, or you notice more benign symptoms that persist for longer than a few days, you must seek medical attention. While it may be healthy to take echinacea if you feel a cold coming on, any serious ailment should be diagnosed by a health care practitioner before undertaking an herbal cure.

Self-diagnosis and self-care are by nature subject to limits. Conventional medicine is best used in crisis situations, and herbs are best used in noncrisis situations.

Professionals can help you avoid treating something that does not exist or failing to treat something that does. Further, health practitioners can help you evaluate the extent of your progress on the herbal regimen. Consultation is especially important if you are taking other medications; while some herbs can work with prescription drugs, others may not. Some herbs can increase the effects of prescription drugs, so you may need a lower dose of their regular medication. Suddenly stopping a prescription medication and/or a drug interaction with herbs can be hazardous to one's health. Pregnant and lactating women should always consult their primary care practitioner before taking any herbal medicines.

You must also have reasonable expectations of herbal medicine: Taking an herb for a few days will not undo ten years of poor health habits, nor is it wise to replace a healthy diet with herbal supplements. If you eat a healthy, varied diet that is high in fresh foods, especially fruits, vegetables, and whole grains, your use of herbal supplements can be targeted on chronic but non-critical ailments.

Sometimes walking into a health food store or pharmacy is highly confusing. Many people are overwhelmed by the wide assortment of products and brands. The following basic guidelines will help when selecting herbal medicines.

Store Clerks Are Not Experts
They do not have an adequate scientific background to counsel people.

Go with a Name Brand
Since the industry is unregulated, it is best to choose products made by large, reputable companies that have been in business for a long time. Many excellent products are produced in Germany and France, where they must meet strict production standards.

Check the Label
Look for the word "standardized," which tells you that the product consistently contains a certain percentage of a specific chemical.

Check to See If the Claims Are Reasonable
Be wary of promises of instant cures for complicated disorders. If something sounds too good to be true, it probably is.

Consider the Product's Form
A liquid, powder, or solid extract is generally best. Bulk herbs can lose their potency quickly. Many herbal tinctures are 50 percent grain alcohol, which may be a problem

for people with a history of alcohol abuse or for those who take drugs that can interact with alcohol.

Be Wary of Ultra-Combination Products

If the product has more than six ingredients, it probably contains a small amount of each. The fact that herbs are combined does not make the product necessarily better. If you need ginkgo to boost your memory, it is better to get it full strength than to get a product diluted with ginseng, garlic, and other herbs.

Take the Right Dose

Do not take higher doses than the label recommends. Exceeding the recommended dose can lead to toxicity. Most herbal remedies are not to be given to children under the age of one unless directed by an experienced practitioner. Children ages 1 to 6 are typically given one-third the adult dose while children ages 6 to 12 receive one-half the adult dose. People over 65 years may need to reduce the dosage also.

Watch for Side Effects

If you have any unusual symptoms, such as allergies, rashes, heart palpitations, or headaches, stop taking the herb immediately and see a health care practitioner.

Give It Time to Work

Evaluate how the product makes you feel. After 30 days, ask yourself whether the product has made a difference in your health. If you are not sure, stop taking the herb to gauge the difference.

Safety First

Inform your primary health care practitioner about the herbal remedies you are taking. Remember that herbal remedies can be risky. Chaparral, sold as teas and pills to fight cancer and "purify blood," has been linked to serious liver damage. Dieter's teas, containing such ingredients as senna, aloe, rhubarb root, buckthorn, cascara, and castor oil, act as laxatives that, when consumed in excessive amounts, can disrupt potassium levels and contribute to cardiac arrhythmias. Ephedra, also called *ma huang*, is an herb used most often for asthma. It is a cardiac and nervous system stimulant containing ephedrine, which can cause anxiety, psychotic episodes, hypertension, stroke, tachycardia, arrhythmias, and cardiac arrest. Mixing ephedra with caffeine or other substances, as the OTC energy-boosting products do, can increase its dangers. Ephedra should not be combined with theophylline, thyroid hormone, tricyclic antidepressants, methylphenidate, or any other drugs that can cause tachycardia or hypertension. Several states have banned supplements containing ephedrine because of the dangers.

If you plan on regularly using herbal remedies, invest in a good herbal reference guide to ensure proper information. One suggestion is James A. Duke's book, *The Green Pharmacy* (Rodale Press, 1997), or Daniel Mowrey's book, *Scientific Validation of Herbal Medicine* (Keats Pub, 1990), or consult with the one of the organizations in the resource list. The U.S. Department of Agriculture provides free access to 80,000 records on herb taxonomy and use of herbs worldwide, developed by Dr. James A. Duke.

Traditional Chinese remedies are taken as an herbal drink. Many Americans, however, complain about the bitter taste and inconvenience of steeping the herbs for hours at a time. Dr. James H. Zhou, formerly a professor at Yale University School of Medicine and founder of HerbaSway, has developed a line of Chinese herbal teas and elixirs in pleasant-tasting liquid concentrates that are becoming more popular among Western consumers.

Getting More Information About Herbal Medicine

The American public is demanding more information about herbal remedies. In the best of all worlds, consumers would have an educated professional—a nurse, a pharmacist, or a doctor—to help guide them through the process of using herbal remedies. That is the situation in Germany, where health care practitioners and pharmacists must be knowledgeable about natural remedies, their approved uses, their potential side effects, and how they should be prescribed. It has not been true in the United States but is sure to change in the near future. Schools of nursing and schools of medicine are including courses on alternative medicine in their curriculum. The College of Pharmacy at the University of Illinois at Chicago has become a collaborating center with the World Health Organization's traditional medicine program and offers a required course in herbal therapy. The resources listed below can also provide good information on selecting an herbal treatment program.

The Absolute Minimum

■ Plants are the original pharmaceuticals. Herbal therapies seek a return to the unprocessed curative properties of plants.

■ Plant components called phytonutrients are believed to be the source of the healing properties of herbs.

■ Herbal preparations can be administered in the form of raw herbs, tinctures, extracts, or even poultices. Care should be taken with all herbal therapies, though, as many plants can have toxic side effects or trigger allergic reactions.

Resources

■ American Botanical Council

www.herbalgram.org

■ American Herbalists Guild

www.americanherbalistsguild.com

■ East/West School of Herbology

www.planetherbs.com

■ FDA Consumer Information Line

www.fda.gov

■ HerbaSway

www.herbasway.com

■ Herb Research Foundation

www.herbs.org

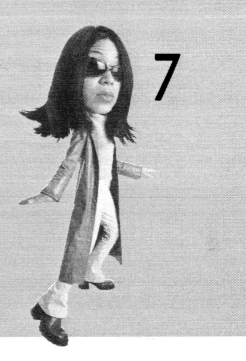

7

NATUROPATHY

Naturopathic medicine is not just a system of medicine but a way of life, with emphasis on client responsibility, patient education, health maintenance, and disease prevention. It may be the model health system of the future, given the movement toward healthy lifestyles, healthy diets, and preventive health care.

What Is Naturopathy?

The basic precepts of naturopathy are similar to those in ancient medical systems throughout the world. Naturopathy can trace its philosophical roots to the Hippocratic school of medicine around 400 BC. Hippocrates had a holistic approach to clients and instructed his students only to prescribe wholesome treatments and avoid causing harm or hurt. Furthermore, Hippocrates thought that the entire universe followed natural laws and the role of the physician was to understand and support nature's own cures.

Naturopathic medicine grew out of the 19th-century medical systems of America and Europe. The term itself was coined by Dr. John Scheel of New York City in 1895, although it was Benedict Lust who formalized naturopathy in 1902 as both a system of medicine and a way of life. By the early 1900s, more than 20 naturopathic schools of medicine were operating in the United States. In the 1920s and 1930s, naturopathic journals encouraged a diet high in fiber and low in red meat, the same type of diet promoted by the National Institutes of Health and the National Cancer Institute in the 1990s. With the development of antibiotics and vaccines in the 1940s and 1950s, the popularity of naturopathy began to decline as people began to rely on these medical breakthroughs. The 1970s saw a renewal in the importance of nutrition, healthy lifestyles, and environmental cleanup programs. This interest continued to grow into what is now the American interest in alternative medicine.

In order for naturopathic medicine to establish itself as a legitimate health care system, it needed to establish accredited schools and conduct credible research. Currently five schools exist in the United States and Canada: Bastyr University in Seattle, Washington; National College of Naturopathic Medicine in Portland, Oregon; the Southwest College of Naturopathic Medicine and Health Science in Scottsdale, Arizona; University of Bridgeport in Connecticut; and the Canadian College of Naturopathic Medicine in Toronto, Ontario. The Council on Naturopathic Medical Education is the accrediting agency for programs in the United States and Canada.

The scope of a naturopathy practice is determined by individual state laws. Currently, 11 states and 5 Canadian provinces issue licenses for naturopathic physicians (NDs). The laws typically allow standard diagnostic procedures, a range of therapies, vaccinations, and limited prescriptive rights. Some states allow the practice of natural childbirth. In states that do not license NDs, anyone can call herself/himself a naturopathic doctor after completing some correspondence courses. These individuals may give seminars and advise people on healthy lifestyles, but they are not permitted to diagnose illness or to prescribe treatment. When seeking a ND as a primary care physician, people you should always ask for verification of graduation from an accredited naturopathic medical school.

The education of naturopathic physicians is extensive and similar to conventional medical education. Four years of medical school follow a college degree in a biological science. The first two years of medical school include courses in anatomy, cell biology, nutrition, physiology, pathology, neurosciences, histology, pharmacology, biostatistics, epidemiology, and public health as well as alternative therapies. Some differences are significant, however. For example, conventional medical students may have only four course hours of nutritional education, while naturopathic medical students have 138 course hours in nutrition. The third and fourth years of medical school are oriented toward clinical experience in diagnosis and treatment. Today's naturopathic doctor is an extensively educated, primary care physician able to utilize a broad range of conventional and alternative therapies.

How Does Naturopathy Work?

Naturopathic medicine holds the same view of human physiology, bodily functions, and disease process as conventional medicine. While many alternative health care professions are defined by the therapies used, naturopathy is defined more by its basic concepts.

Healing Power of Nature

Naturopathic theory holds that the body innately knows how to maintain health and heal itself. Natural laws of life operate inside and outside the body and the physician's job is to support and restore them by using techniques and medicines that are in harmony with the natural processes. These natural methods are geared to strengthen the body's own healing ability. Faith, hope, and beliefs may be the most significant aspects of any treatment. Many studies have documented the ability of the mind to affect the process of disease, either positively or negatively. Physicians consider issues such as "What does it mean, for this person, to be in balance?" and "What are the healing powers available for this person?"

First, Do No Harm

Iatrogenic illness, the creation of additional illness as a result of medical treatment, is a major health problem in the United States. A 1981 study found that at least one-third of all inpatients suffered some ill effect from the medical treatment plan. Nine percent of the patients experienced a life threatening or permanently disabling complication, and two percent of patients died from the iatrogenic disorder. Recent studies have found that adverse drug reactions appear to be between the fourth and sixth leading cause of death in the United States. Furthermore, drug-related injuries occur in almost seven percent of hospitalized patients.

As Hippocrates said, "Above all else, do no harm." Naturopathic physicians prefer noninvasive treatments that minimize the risk of harmful side effects, and always take care to consider questions like "Will a delay in treatment be of benefit?" and "What is the potential for harm with this particular treatment plan?"

Find the Cause

Naturopathic physicians look for the underlying causes of disease and try to help patients get rid of them. These causes are often found in people's lifestyles, habits, and/or diets. Physical, mental, emotional, and spiritual factors are important in determining cause. Issues to be considered are "What are the causative factors contributing to 'dis-ease' in this person? Of these causative factors, which are avoidable or preventable? What are the limiting factors in this person's life?"

Physician as Teacher

The word doctor comes from the Latin *docere*, meaning to teach. Unlike many conventional medical physicians who have little time to teach, the primary focus of naturopathic physicians is teaching people how to achieve health and avoid disease. The emphasis is on people learning to assume responsibility for themselves and their well-being. People increasingly realize that their good health is dependent to a great extent on treating their bodies properly. People are looking for health care practitioners who can teach them how to treat all aspects in a healthy manner. Naturopathic physicians are an appropriate choice for many—especially if you've asked yourself questions like "What type of patient education is my physician providing? In what ways does my physician encourage and support me being responsible for my health and well-being?"

Health Comes from Within

Naturopathy views health as more than the absence of disease. Health is a dynamic process that allows people to thrive despite various internal and external stresses. Health arises from a complex interaction of physical, mental, emotional, spiritual, dietary, genetic, environmental, lifestyle, and other components. Health is characterized by positive emotions, thoughts, and actions. Healthy people are energetic and creative as they live goal-directed lives. Health does not come from doctors, pills, or surgery, but rather from people's own efforts to take appropriate care of themselves.

Naturopathic physicians recognize the role of bacteria and viruses in illness but view these as secondary factors. They believe that most disease is the direct result of ignoring natural laws. These violations include eating processed foods, having little exercise and rest, living a fast-paced lifestyle, focusing on negative thoughts and emotions, and being exposed to environmental toxins. Disease-promoting habits lead people away from optimal function toward progressively greater dysfunction in body, mind, and spirit. Naturopathy recognizes death is inevitable, but believes progressive disability is often avoidable.

Naturopathic Diagnosis and Treatment

Naturopathic physicians practice as primary care providers. They see people of all ages suffering from all types of disorders and diseases. They make conventional medical diagnoses using standard diagnostic procedures such as physical examinations, laboratory tests, and radiology. They also perform a detailed assessment of lifestyle, looking for physical, emotional, dietary, genetic, environmental, and family dynamics contributing to a disorder. Since health or disease is a complex interaction of factors, naturopathic physicians treat the whole person, taking all these elements into account. Careful attention to each person's individuality and susceptibility to disease is critical to accurate diagnosis. When necessary, naturopathic physicians, like family practice physicians, refer patients to other health care professionals for hospitalization, surgery, or other specialized care.

Naturopathic physicians do not provide emergency care nor do they do major surgery. They rarely prescribe drugs and they treat clients in private practice and outpatient clinics, not in hospitals. Some physicians practice natural childbirth at home or in a clinic.

The therapeutic approach of the naturopathic doctor is to help people heal themselves and to use opportunities to guide and educate people in developing healthier lifestyles. The goal of treatment is the restoration of health and normal body function, rather than the application of a particular therapy. Naturopathic doctors use virtually every natural medical therapy described in this text.

Naturopathic physicians mix and match different approaches, customizing treatment for each person. The least invasive intervention to support the body's natural healing processes is a primary consideration. These interventions include dietetics, therapeutic nutrition, herbs (European, Native American, and Chinese), physical therapy, spinal manipulation, acupuncture, lifestyle counseling, stress management, exercise therapy, homeopathy, and hydrotherapy.

Counseling is an important intervention because mental, emotional, and spiritual factors are part of the holistic approach. Lifestyle modification is crucial to the success of naturopathy. While it is relatively easy to tell a person to stop smoking, get more exercise, and reduce stress, such lifestyle changes are often difficult for people to make. The naturopathic physician is educated to assist people in making the needed changes. This process involves helping people acknowledge the need to change habits; identifying triggers for unhealthy habits; setting realistic and progressive goals; establishing a support group of family, friends, and others with similar difficulties; and giving people positive recognition for their gains.

THE ABSOLUTE MINIMUM

- Naturopathy was developed in the U.S. in the early 20th century, but the basis for its beliefs lie in the ancient Greek Hippocratic school.
- Naturopathy believes that health and healing lie within all of us, and that living in harmony with nature will yield a long and healthy life.
- Naturopathic doctors help people heal themselves and use opportunities to guide and educate people in developing healthier lifestyles.

RESOURCES

- American Association of Naturopathic Physicians

  www.naturopathic.org
- British Naturopathy Association

  www.naturopaths.org.uk

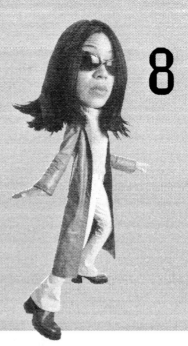

8

HOMEOPATHY

Homeopathy is derived from the Greek words *omoios*, meaning "similar" and *pathos* meaning "feeling." It is a self-healing system, assisted by small doses of remedies or medicines, which is useful in a variety of acute and chronic disorders. The practice of homeopathy in the United States has increased tremendously since the 1980s, corresponding to the increase in other forms of alternative medicine. Homeopathic medicine is practiced worldwide, especially in Europe, Latin America, and Asia. In Great Britain, visits to homeopaths are increasing at a rate of 29% a year. Forty-two percent of British physicians refer people to homeopaths. Forty percent of Dutch physicians, 25 percent of German physicians, and 32% of French physicians use homeopathy. India has more than 100 homeopathic medical colleges and more than 100,000 homeopathic practitioners.

What Is Homeopathy?

Homeopathy as a therapeutic system is approximately 200 years old. It was developed by Samuel Hahnemann (1755–1843), a German physician and chemist. Homeopathy came to most of Europe, the United States, Russia, and Latin America in the 1830s. During epidemics of cholera, typhus, and scarlet fever, homeopathy was significantly more effective than the conventional medical approaches of the times. In 1869, the American Institute of Homeopathy opened free dispensaries for the poor and voted to admit female physicians, unheard of in conventional medicine. By the 1890s, 15% of American physicians used some homeopathic remedies in their practice, learned in the 22 homeopathic medical schools and practiced in more than 100 homeopathic hospitals.

note

In the U.S., the homeopathic drug market has grown into a multimillion dollar industry. The National Center for Homeopathy estimates that Americans spend $165 million a year for homeopathic preparations, and that sales are rising by 20–25 percent a year. Most of these remedies are not regulated by the FDA and are available as over-the-counter medications.

During and after the Civil War, the practice of medicine began to change with technical achievements such as anesthesia, antiseptics, surgery, microbiology, vaccines, and antibiotics. State legislatures began to license physicians and accredit medical schools. The American Medical Association (AMA) invited homeopaths to become members in exchange for licensing, seeking to create a monopoly against lay healers, midwives, and herbalists. When the homeopaths chose not to join forces, the AMA began to persecute homeopathy, and in 1914, proposed uniform standards of medical education and assumed the power of accreditation, using it to phase out homeopathic colleges. Most homeopathic medical schools closed down, and by the 1930s others had converted to conventional medical schools.

The Homeopathic Pharmacopoeia of the United States was written into federal law in 1938 under the Federal Food, Drug, and Cosmetic Act, making the manufacture and sale of homeopathic medicines legal in this country. In the 1960s, homeopathy's popularity began to revive in the United States. According to a 1999 survey of Americans and their health, over 6 million Americans had used homeopathy in the preceding 12 months.

About half of the homeopaths in the United States are physicians. The others are licensed health care practitioners such as nurse practitioners, dentists, naturopathic physicians, chiropractors, acupuncturists, and veterinarians. Training in homeopathy is offered through professional courses at the National Center for Homeopathy in Alexandria, Virginia. The certification process involves a specified number of hours of training, three years of clinical practice, and written and oral examinations. Certification earns the right to place the designation "DIIt" after one's name. Licensure to practice homeopathy varies among the states. At the present time, five states—Arizona, Connecticut, Delaware, Nevada, and New Hampshire—have medical boards regulating homeopaths. Other states regulate practitioners through the "scope of practice" guidelines issued by medical boards.

How Does Homeopathy Work?

At first glance, Homeopathy might seem absurd: treating an illness with a tiny quantity of the substance that caused the illness in the first place. This first glance would, however, be a very superficial assessment of the system Dr. Hahnemann developed, as we shall see.

Law of Similars

Hahnemann proposed the use of the Law of Similars, which claims that a natural substance that produces a given symptom in a healthy person can cure it in a sick person. The substance that causes symptoms most closely resembling the illness being treated is the one most likely to initiate a curative response for that person. Hence the name homeopathy: "similar feeling."

By definition, the natural compounds used in homeopathy will produce symptoms of disease, if taken in large amounts. In the doses used by homeopaths, however, these remedies stimulate a person's self-healing capacity. As the well-known alternative doctor and author Andrew Weil states, "The difference between a poison and a medicine is the dose." An example is seen in the use of ipecac, which in large doses causes severe nausea and vomiting. Women who are experiencing the nausea and vomiting of pregnancy, however, can use small doses of Ipecac to cure those same symptoms. The most extreme example is, of course, chemotherapy, where the patient is effectively poisoned in an attempt to halt the uncontrolled cell growth that would otherwise kill them.

Law of Infinitesimals

Natural healing compounds are specially prepared for homeopathic use through a process of serial dilution. The compound is first dissolved in a water-alcohol mixture called the "mother tincture." One drop of the tincture is then mixed with 10 drops of water-alcohol, and this process is repeated hundreds or thousands of times depending on the potency being prepared. At each step of the dilution, the vial is vigorously shaken, called *succussion*, which seems to be an essential step. The homeopathic belief is that the more the substance is diluted, the more potent it becomes as a remedy.

The remedies are diluted beyond the point at which any molecules of the substance can theoretically still be found in the solution. This paradox, that the remedy becomes more potent through dilution, and the fact that the exact mechanism that makes a homeopathic cure work is unknown, is the reason many biomedical scientists reject homeopathic medicine. Of course, if biomedical pharmacologists had to understand exactly how the conventional drugs they develop worked, our pharmacopoeia would likely be much smaller.

A number of theories are proposed for homeopathy's effectiveness. A remedy may be like a hologram: No matter how many times a substance is diluted, a smaller but complete essence of the substance remains. Modern chaos theory supports the observation that major changes occur in living organisms when bodily substances are activated only slightly. The basic assumption of chaos theory is that minute changes can have huge effects. Advances in quantum physics have led some scientists to suggest that electromagnetic energy in the remedies interact with the body on some level.

Researchers in physical chemistry have proposed the memory of water theory, which posits that the structure of the water-alcohol solution is altered during the process of dilution and retains its new structure even after the substance is no longer present. It seems likely that remedies work through some bioenergic or subatomic mechanism that we are not yet capable of understanding. The situation may be likened to the products of many of our advances in the understanding of energy, such as radio, television, microwave ovens, and cordless telephones, all of which were previously unimaginable.

When Life Is Out of Balance

Homeopathy is a method for treating the sick rather than a set of hypotheses about the nature of health and illness. The assumption is, however, that a vital force—known as qi or prana in other traditions—exists. It is necessary to have adequate nutrition, exercise, rest, good hygiene, and a healthy environment to adapt and maintain homeostasis. In other words, health is the ability of people to adapt their equilibrium in response to internal and external change. Illness is primarily a disturbance of the vital force, manifested as symptoms of distress. Vital force or life energy is the ultimate origin of health and illness alike, ending only with the death of the person.

Symptoms of illness represent people's attempts to heal themselves. Thus, homeopathy views symptoms as an adaptive reaction that is the best possible response that can be made in the present circumstances. For example, a cough is the body's attempt to clear the bronchi; inflammation is the body's effort to wall off and burn out invading foreign bodies; and fever is the body's way to create an internal environment that is less conducive to bacterial or viral growth. Given this perspective, the therapeutic approach is to aid the body's efforts to adapt to stress or infection.

Thus, for someone with a high fever, homeopaths may recommend belladonna, which increases the natural healing response of body heat.

The Law of Similars is a stimulation of immune and defense responses, leading to spontaneous resolution of symptoms as the illness is conquered. In like manner, two of the few conventional therapies that seek to stimulate the body's own healing reaction, immunization and allergy treatment, have the homeopathic Law of Similars as their basis. Other applications in conventional medicine include the use of radiation in the treatment of cancer and Ritalin in the treatment of hyperactive children. The majority of interventions in conventional medicine, however, attempt to oppose symptoms by exerting a greater and opposite force. Medicines are designed to "cure" by suppressing symptoms such as the use of aspirin in an effort to control or limit people's fevers. The danger is that, over time, suppressive treatments may actually strengthen disease processes instead of resolving them.

A Holistic Diagnosis

Homeopathic diagnosis is a holistic and detailed process—the initial assessment may last several hours. Practitioners assess the whole person, looking at every aspect of physical, emotional, and mental life. A multitude of factors are considered, such as nutritional status, emotional imbalance, and environmental stress. It is believed that no part can be isolated from the whole person.

The homeopathic interview itself is a powerful healing experience because clients are encouraged to tell their story in its entirety. They are encouraged to speak for as long a time as possible. This process of sharing pain and suffering begins the healing process. During the interview, the practitioner observes everything about the person including posture, dress, facial expression, tone of voice, rate of speech, and so forth.

The physical exam is a head-to-toe assessment with the inclusion of laboratory work as needed to establish a diagnosis. Answers to questions are elicited in an attempt to fully understand the significance of the symptoms:

- Subjective symptoms such as pain, vertigo, fatigue, or anger
- Localization of symptoms such as one-sided, wandering, radiating, or diffuse
- Factors that modify the symptoms, making them better or worse, such as time of day, hot or cold, weather, diet, or emotional state
- Quality of symptoms such as burning, aching, throbbing
- Rate of onset or resolution of the symptoms such as sudden or gradual
- Symptoms that appear simultaneously or in sequence

Symptoms are classified into three categories—the general physical symptoms, the local symptoms, and the mental and emotional symptoms. General physical symptoms include such things as sleep, appetite, energy, temperature, or generalized bodily pain. Local symptoms occur in particular parts of the body such as swelling in the right elbow or pain in the left leg. Included in local symptoms are those related to a specific organ function such as shortness of breath or palpitations. Mental and emotional symptoms include anxiety, irritability, anger, tearfulness, isolation, or suspiciousness. This composite picture of the person is far more important than any isolated laboratory findings or abstract disease category in formulating the diagnosis. Homeopathic practitioners do not hesitate to refer to biomedical specialists for conventional drugs or surgery.

Take Two Drops and Call Me in the Morning: Homeopathic Treatment

As in other complementary practices, the initial question is always "Who is the person?" rather than "What is the disease?" This focus ensures an individualized approach to treatment. Each person with the same presenting complaint may be treated with different remedies, depending on the totality of physical, mental, and emotional symptoms. A person with a sore throat may be prescribed one of six or seven common remedies for sore throats, depending on whether the pain is worse on the right or left side, what time of day it is worse, how thirst and appetite are affected, and the individual's emotional state.

The science and the art of homeopathy are to find the remedy with the ability to mimic most closely the sick person's pattern of symptoms. Practitioners use only one remedy at a time, since administering different remedies for different symptoms makes it difficult to know which remedy was effective. Not only are the smallest possible doses used, typically only one dose is given, which allows time for the remedy to complete its action without further interference. If necessary, a dose may be repeated or another remedy may be tried. A temporary worsening of the symptoms may occur after receiving the remedy, which is usually mild and short-lived and may be an indication that the correct remedy was chosen.

Homeopathy is used to treat both acute and chronic health problems as well as for health promotion. It cannot cure conditions resulting from structural, long-term, organic changes such as cirrhosis, diabetes, chronic obstructive lung disease, advanced neurological diseases, or cancer. In some of these cases, however, homeopathy can relieve the symptoms and increase the patient's comfort level.

Traumatic injuries affect nearly everyone in similar ways and thus the remedies are fairly standard. Epidemic infectious diseases also tend to affect most victims in the same way and individuals are usually treated with the same remedy. Common infectious illnesses such as urinary tract infections, respiratory infections, or ear infections demonstrate more individual symptoms and require more individualization in selecting the remedy. Chronic illness such as ulcerative colitis, rheumatoid arthritis, asthma, and skin disorders are considered to be constitutional. Thus these disorders require the most skillful assessment, individualized prescription, and follow-up.

The Homeopathic Pharmacopoeia of the United States, listing more than 2,000 remedies, is the official standard for preparation and prescription. Most remedies come from plants used in traditional herbal medicine. A few remedies come from animal sources and others from naturally occurring chemical compounds. Table 8.1 lists examples of remedies. Some, such as mercury and belladonna, would be poisonous in large doses but are safe in the superdiluted homeopathic doses. These remedies rank among the safest medicines available.

Table 8.1 Examples of Homeopathic Remedies

Vegetable	Mineral	Animal
Herbs: comfrey, eyebright, mullein, yellow dock	Metals: copper, gold, lead, tin, zinc	Venoms: jellyfish, insects, spiders, mollusks, crustaceans, fish, snakes, amphibians
Foods and spices: cayenne, garlic, mustard,onion	Salts: calcium sulfate, sodium chloride, potassium carbonate	Secretions: ambergris, musk, cuttlefish ink
Fragrances, resins, residues: amber, petroleum, charcoal, creosote	Acids: hydrochloric, nitric, phosphoric, sulfuric	Milks
		Hormones
Mushrooms, lichens, mosses	Elemental substances: carbon, hydrogen, iodine, phosphorus, sulfur	Glandular and Tissue Extracts
	Constituents of earth's crust: silica, aluminum oxide, ores, rocks, lavas, mineral waters	Disease Products: vaccines, abcesses, tuberculosis, gonorrhea, syphilis

How Do I Get Started with Homeopathy?

People who are interested in homeopathic remedies can find low potency remedies in health food stores. Higher potency remedies are obtained from homeopathic pharmaceutical companies under the direction of experienced homeopathic practitioners. Since remedies are inactivated by direct sunlight and heat, you must store the preparations in a cool, dark, dry place, away from other strong-smelling substances. When taking a remedy, you should have nothing by mouth for at least 30 minutes before and after the dose. Many homeopaths discourage the use of coffee, mint, camphor, and other strongly aromatic substances while undergoing treatment, since such substances may reverse the effects of the remedy. Camphor is a component in chest rubs as well as in many cosmetics, skin creams, and lip balms. If the remedy is in the form of a pellet, it should be held under the tongue and allowed to dissolve slowly. If the remedy is a liquid, it is held in the mouth for 1 to 2 minutes before swallowing.

Prescription medications, especially those given for potentially life-threatening disorders such as asthma, should not be stopped abruptly when beginning homeopathic care. As you improve, your prescribing physician may advise a gradual decrease in dosage, but you should not undertake such a reduction on your own. Acupuncture and chiropractic medicine should not be started at the same time as homeopathic remedies, but if already instituted, may be continued.

A number of homeopathic remedies can be used to speed recovery and prevent recurrences of acute conditions such as colds, stomachaches, coughs, and headaches. Although many remedies are used for conditions that subside on their own, they can dramatically speed recovery and often prevent recurrences. Since homeopathic medicines are considerably safer than conventional drugs, it often makes sense to use them as the first resort and to consider using conventional drugs if the homeopathic remedies work too slowly or not at all. You should read all the information on the label to select the right remedy. If it says, for example, that the remedy is best used when the symptoms appear suddenly, then that remedy is not likely to be effective for a condition that emerged almost unnoticed over several days. Keep these three guidelines in mind when considering the use of homeopathic remedies:

- The more the better—that is, the more the symptoms match that of the remedy, the more likely it will work.
- The less the better: The more diluted the remedy, the more powerful it is.
- It's working if you feel better within 24 hours. If not, you may have the wrong remedy and may need a different remedy or may need to see a health care practitioner.

Many people keep homeopathic remedies on hand and ready to use. Table 8.2 lists the top 10 remedies that help with the most common physical problems and emotional difficulties.

Table 8.2 Homeopathic Treatments to Try

Treatment	Indications
Bryonia (wild hops	for coughs that are worsened by simple breathing; headaches that are increased by bending over, walking, or even moving the eyes; constipation with dry, hard stools.
Allium cepa (onion)	for colds or respiratory allergies where symptoms resemble the reaction of a person exposed to the mist of an onion: watery eyes, clear nasal discharge, and sneezes, all of which are aggravated by exposure to heat.
Pulsatilla (windflower)	need is based on the type of person, rather than a specific ailment. Helpful for people who are highly emotional, weepy, impressionable, easily influenced, fearful of abandonment, and worried about what others think of them. May also be used for digestive disorders, allergies, earaches, headaches, insomnia, and PMS.
Ignatia (St. Ignatius bean)	for people who experience anxiety or grief.
Arsenicum album (arsenic)	used for many conditions especially when symptoms are worse after midnight, when burning symptoms are predominant, when great thirst occurs, or when the person is high strung and restless.
Belladonna (deadly nightshade)	for fevers or inflammation that begin rapidly, with a red or flushed appearance, and the person is hypersensitive to touch or light.
Gelsemium (yellow jessamine)	for classic flu symptoms accompanied by lack of thirst. Helpful for headaches in the back part of the head.
Nux vomica (poison nut)	useful after overdosing with food or drink, indigestion, constipation, and headaches that are worse at night and on waking.
Aconitum (monkshood)	for colds, flu, coughs, and sore throats with rapid onset.
Rhus toxicodendron (poison ivy)	helpful for arthritis syndromes, flu, sprains and strains, and sore throats. For people who feel pain on initial motion that eases with continued motion and symptoms worsen in cold or wet weather.

THE ABSOLUTE MINIMUM

- Homeopathy treatment is based on the administration of minutely small amounts of naturally occurring substances that, in large quantities, would cause the illness being treated.

- The preparation of homeopathic remedies is highly involved and precise; more than 2000 distinct compounds are available.

- More than half of the homeopaths in the U.S. are medical doctors; the practice of homeopathy alongside conventional medicine is even more common in Europe.

RESOURCES

- American Institute of Homeopathy

  www.homeopathyusa.org

- Homeopathic Educational Services

  www.homeopathic.com

- National Center for Homeopathy

  www.homeopathic.org

- NIH Report on Homeopathy

  nccam.nih.gov/health/homeopathy/

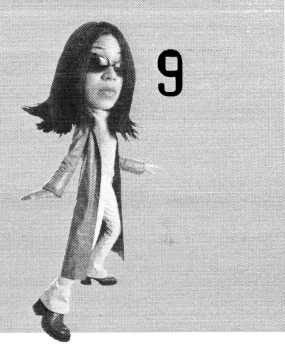

9

AROMATHERAPY

Aromatherapy is the therapeutic use of the essential oils of plants. The chemicals found in the essential oils are absorbed into the body, resulting in physiological or psychological benefit. Aromatherapy uses essential oils to treat symptoms and as such has no theory of health and illness or a system of diagnosis.

What Is Aromatherapy?

Scientists have long known that certain scents have the power to evoke strong physical and emotional reactions but rarely has that knowledge been used in conventional medicine. Healthy humans can smell as many as 10,000 different odors, ranging from the deep fragrance of jasmine to the putrid stench of sewage. Most people, however, do not realize how much the sense of smell affects their daily lives.

Aromatherapy has been forgotten and ignored for many years but is now one of the fastest growing alternative therapies in Europe and the United States. The term aromatherapy has become more than a buzzword since the mid 1980s. In the United States, it is now a generic term in the public domain and, as such, it cannot be trademarked by an individual or business.

Essential oils come from all over the world—lavender from France, sandalwood and jasmine from India, rose from Turkey and Bulgaria, geranium from the island of Reunion, eucalyptus and tea tree from Australia, and mint from the United States. Today, only 3% of essential oils are used in therapy; the remaining 97% are used in the perfume and cosmetic industry. With increased popularity, aromatherapy has become a $300 million-a-year market in the United States.

The History of Aromatherapy

Almost all ancient cultures recognized the value of aromatic plants in maintaining health. Ancient Egyptians used scented oils daily to soften and protect their skin from the harsh, dry climate. They created various fragrances for personal benefit as well as for use in rituals and ceremonies. Fragrances were considered a part of the personal purification necessary to reach a realm of higher spirituality. Oils were dispersed into the air to purify the environment and provide protection from evil spirits. Egyptians were the first to perfect embalming with the use of aromatic plants and oils.

Priests and physicians used oils thousands of years before the time of Christ. The Romans diffused oils in their temples and political buildings and bathed in hot tubs scented with oils. Ancient Arabian people studied the chemistry of plants and developed the process of distillation for extraction of essential oils. Throughout Asia perfumes were prized for both medicinal and cosmetic properties. Hundreds of references are made to oils in the Bible such as frankincense, myrrh, and cinnamon. Many were used as protection against disease and for anointing and healing the sick. Hippocrates, the father of Western medicine, reportedly said, "The way to health is to have an aromatic bath and scented massage every day." Sounds like good advice to us.

In the 12th century, trade routes from the Middle East brought spices, herbs, and exotic scents to Europe, leading to the compilation of many books on therapeutic plant remedies. In the Americas, shamans also used herbs and aromatics in the bathing of patients to transform their energy field. Smoke from plants was often blown over patients as part of the healing ceremony.

Not Just for Perfume Anymore

Although oils were used with great effectiveness in ancient times, they were largely forgotten by the Western world until resurrected in the twentieth century by a French cosmetic chemist, Maurice-Rene Cattefosse. While working in his laboratory in 1920, he had an accident that resulted in a third degree burn of his hand and forearm. He plunged his arm into a vat of lavender oil, thinking that it was water. To his surprise, the burning stopped within a few moments. With the continual application of lavender oil over the next few weeks, the burn healed completely without a trace of a scar. This incident was the beginning of Cattefosse's fascination with the therapeutic properties of essential oils. He carried out experiments using oils to cure burns, treat wounds, and prevent gangrene and in 1937 coined the term *aromatherapie*.

Since the 1980s, numerous schools of massage and aromatherapy have opened in Britain. Training in aromatherapy has grown, and courses in it are part of the nursing degree program in some nursing colleges and universities. Aromatherapists practice in a number of settings including private practices, general medical clinics, and hospitals. Currently, no law specifies a minimum level of training and practice in the United Kingdom.

Some people in the United States, after a weekend course, call themselves "aromatherapists." They may know little about plant chemistry and the specific ways in which the oils need to be formulated. Their self-proclaimed title is fine if they use oils only for fragrance and perfume. Using oil formulas for a specific therapeutic action is inappropriate, however, for individuals with this limited knowledge. The Institute of Aromatherapy in Denville, New Jersey, was approved in 1997 by the New Jersey Department of Education, making it the first state-approved aromatherapy school in the United States. Their 200 in-class hours are designed to provide a comprehensive knowledge of aromatherapy including classes in botany, psychoneuroimmunology, and plant chemistry.

How Does Aromatherapy Work?

The delivery of aromatherapuetic treatment begins with the extraction of essential oils from plants. The oils are then matched to the patient's specific concerns and needs, and the oil, or more typically a blend of oils, is then delivered in a way that will most directly address the patient's concern.

Essential Oils

Essential oils are volatile liquids that are distilled or cold pressed from plants. Although chemically they are oils and as such do not mix with water, the term oil is somewhat misleading, since they feel like water rather than oil. Varying amounts of essential oil can be extracted from a particular plant, which influences the price of the oil. For example, it takes 220 pounds of rose petals to furnish less than two ounces of the essential oil. Other plants such as lavender or eucalyptus give a much greater proportion. One half ounce of rose oil may cost $200 while the same amount of orange oil may cost only a few dollars. Table 9.1 shows the many different plants parts from which oils are extracted.

Table 9.1   Waste Not, Want Not: Plant Parts That Yield Essential Oils

Plant Part	Oils Extracted
Leaves	Eucalyptus, peppermint
Flowers	Lavender, rose
Blossoms	Orange, neroli
Fruits	Lemon, mandarin
Grasses	Lemongrass
Wood	Camphor, sandalwood
Barks	Cinnamon
Gum	Frankincense
Bulbs	Garlic, onion
Dried flower buds	Clove

Essential oils are stored in tiny pockets between plant cell walls. As the plant releases the oil, it circulates through the plant and sends messages that help it function efficiently. Oils activate and regulate such activities as cellular metabolism, photosynthesis, and cellular respiration. They may also trigger immune responses to assist in coping with stressful changes in the environment and climate. Some oils protect the plant from predators, especially microorganisms, and in so doing are essentially antibacterial, antiviral, and antifungal. Some oils protect the plant by repelling harmful insects while others attract insects or animals that are useful for propagation.

Plant oils are highly concentrated, and it is important to respect their power. One drop of oil is the medical equivalent of one ounce of the parent plant material used in herbal medicine. Essential oils are chemically diverse and may contain a mixture of more than 100 organic compounds including esters, alcohols, aldehydes, ketones, phenols, acids, and so on. Each kind of oil may contain more of some compounds than others, which gives the oil its particular therapeutic use. Table 9.2 lists some of the major chemical components and their therapeutic effects.

Table 9.2   Chemical Compounds of Essential Oils and Their Therapeutic Actions

Compound	Therapeutic Action
Aldehydes	Anti-infectious, boost immune system, sedative
Eugenol	Antiseptic, stimulant
Ketones	Sedative, liquefy mucous, stimulate cell regeneration
Phenols	Antiseptic
Esters	Antispasmodic, calming
Sesquiterpenes	Antihistamines, anti-inflammatory
Acids	Anti-infectious, boost immune system
Oxides	Expectorant, antiparasitic
C10 terpenes	Antiseptic

How Essential Oils Work

Stimulating the sense of smell is, naturally, the primary effect of aromatherapy. The nose contains 5 million smell-sensing cells that allow people to consciously register smells. Each cell has 6–12 hairlike receptors (cilia) that hang down into the stream of air rushing into the nose. These olfactory receptors are the only sensory pathways that open directly to the brain. The cilia detect scents and the nerve cells relay this information directly to the limbic system triggering memories and influencing behavior. The amygdala of the limbic system, which stores and releases emotional memories, is most sensitive to odor or fragrance. Thus, the sense of smell can evoke powerful memories in a split second and change people's perceptions and behaviors.

Also inside the human nose is a small cavity called the *vomero nasal organ (VMO)*, which is lined with a cell type that is unlike any other cell in the human body. The VMO is far less prominent in people than in animals who depend more heavily on smell for guidance. Pheromones are chemical substances produced by one animal that cause a specific reaction in another, usually of the same species, through smell.

The VMO appears to specialize in detecting pheromones without people's conscious awareness. In other words, people do not "smell" pheromones in the same way they smell freshly baked apple pies or essential oils. The scent, however, is registered at some brain level and people respond to it emotionally and/or physically. Many aromatherapeutic compounds are thought to stimulate the VMO.

Olfactory stimulation can trigger negative responses such as intense fear or panic or positive feelings with increased release of endorphins and neurotransmitter (see Table 9.3). Odors stimulate the pituitary gland and hypothalamus and thus impact the production of hormones that control appetite, insulin production, body temperature, metabolism, stress levels, and sex drive. Unlike vision and hearing, the sense of smell is fully functional at birth. Newborns can recognize their mothers by smell, and this sensory response is an important part of bonding. In adult relationships, the sense of smell has a significant role in sensual and sexual attraction.

Table 9.3 Blending Oils According to Effect

Desired Effect	Appropriate Oils
Soothing	Chamomile
Uplifting	Black pepper, coriander, jasmine, juniper, eucalyptus, peppermint, tea tree
Balancing	Cypress, lavender
Uplifting and Soothing	Basil, bergamot, frankincense, ginger, neroli, orange, patchouli, sandalwood
Uplifting and Stimulating	Cedarwood, lemon, lemon grass, myrrh, pine, rose, rosemary, ylang ylang
Uplifting and Balancing	Clary sage, geranium

Examples of Blends

Basil, lavender

Bergamot, cypress, jasmine

Chamomile, lavender

Clary sage, lavender, sandalwood

Eucalyptus, chamomile, lavender, bergamot

Geranium, bergamot, lemon, lavender

Ginger, lavender, orange, neroli

Jasmine, rose, lemon, black pepper

Juniper, bergamot, geranium, frankincense

Lemon, tea tree, ylang ylang

Pine, eucalyptus, lavender

Patchouli, bergamot, geranium

Peppermint, lavender

Bandalwood, ylang ylang, black pepper, neroli

Delivering Essential Oils

In addition to stimulating our scent-detecting organs, and through them the central nervous system, inhaled oil molecules enter the respiratory system. There the molecules attach to oxygen molecules and circulate through the body, bringing with them the potential for activating self-healing processes. The equivalent in conventional medicine is the use of inhalers in the treatment of asthma. Essential oils can be inhaled directly or mixed with a carrier oil. Electrical and fan-assisted equipment or an aromatherapy light bulb ring may be used to scent a room for therapeutic purposes or to simply make the environment more pleasant. Steam inhalers can be used in the treatment of respiratory infections.

Applied externally, essential oils can calm inflamed or irritated skin, soothe sore muscles, decrease muscular tension, and release muscle spasms. Molecules of essential oils are so tiny they are quickly absorbed through the skin and enter the intercellular fluid and the circulatory system, bringing healing nutrients to the cells. Some oils such as basil, tea tree, and thyme encourage the production of white blood cells, while others such as lavender and eucalyptus fight harmful bacteria, viruses, and fungi. Oils may be applied just about anywhere: neck, face, wrists, over the heart, back, arms, legs, and feet. Massage therapists and acupuncturists often use essential oils in their treatments. Benefits are gained not only from the penetration of the oil through the skin but also from inhalation of the vapor and from direct massage of the skin and muscles. Essential oils do not remain in the body and are excreted in urine, feces, perspiration, and exhalation usually in 3–6 hours.

A diffuser is a special air pump designed to disburse the oils in a micro-fine vapor into the atmosphere where they stay suspended for several hours. Diffusing releases oxygenating molecules as well as antiviral, antibacterial, and antiseptic properties. Unlike commercial air fresheners, which mask odors, essential oils clean the air by altering the structure of the molecules that create an unpleasant smell. Essential oils help remove dust particles out of the air and, when diffused in the room, can be an effective air filtration system.

How Can I Get Started with Aromatherapy?

Essential oils influence health on physical, mental, and emotional levels. They have the ability to penetrate cell walls and transport oxygen and nutrients to the cell. Many have antiviral, antibacterial, antifungal, and antiseptic properties. This property of oils may be significant in the future as microbes continue to mutate and develop resistance to known medications. Aromatherapy can be used for the following purposes:

- Prompt the body and mind to function more efficiently
- Decrease and manage stress
- Refresh or recharge oneself
- Regulate moods—some are energizing and some are sedating
- Aid restful sleep
- Act as a first aid measure
- Reduce weight
- Boost the immune system
- Minimize the discomforts of illness and speed recovery
- Refresh room environment

The purity and authenticity of essential oils is critical to their effectiveness. Oils that are diluted, adulterated, or synthetic should not be used for aromatherapy. Those identified as commercial grade essential oils are likely to be diluted or adulterated in some way. Some are diluted with chemical carriers and passed on to the consumer as "pure essential oils" and are found in bath and cosmetic shops. Those labeled as "infused oils" are also adulterated. "Nature identical" oils are synthetic petrochemical-based products. They have been developed to closely mimic the smell and composition of essential oils. They are not identical, however, and lack many of the healing components of essential oils. Other names for synthetic oils are aroma-chemicals, perfume oils, and fragrance oils. Manufacturers have no restrictions on how essential oils are labeled. In general, those described with terms such as genuine, authentic, or premium are more likely to be pure essential oils. Informed consumers read labels carefully and buy from reputable dealers. The Institute of Aromatherapy can provide information on purchasing essential oils.

BE CAREFUL!

Essential oils must not be ingested, since even modest amounts can be fatal, and they must be kept away from children and pets. Pregnant women and persons with epilepsy should consult a knowledgeable health care practitioner or qualified aromatherapist prior to the use of essential oils. Oils other than lavender or tea tree oil must always be diluted before applying on the skin. People who have sensitive skin or allergies should take extra care in massaging the oils into the skin or inhaling the essential oil aromas, and everyone must be careful not to rub their eyes if they have any essential oil on their hands.

Several oils are photosensitive or phototoxic, causing severe sunburn if people are exposed to the sun within six hours after application. These oils include clove, bergamot, angelica, verbena, bitter/sweet orange, lemon, lime, and mandarin. Certain oils have high toxicity levels, and their use should be limited to qualified aromatherapists. These oils include boldo leaf, calamus, yellow camphor, horse-radish, rue, sassafras, savin, tansy, wintergreen, wormseed, and wormwood.

Essential oils are quite potent and can irritate the skin, so they should be diluted with a carrier oil before being used on the skin. Carrier oils contain vitamins, proteins, and minerals that provide added nutrients to the body. Some carrier oils can be purchased at supermarkets, while others may be available only at health food stores. Carrier oils include apricot kernel oil, sunflower oil, soy oil, sweet almond oil, grapeseed oil, sesame oil, avocado oil, jojoba oil, and wheat-germ oil. The fragrance does not have to be intense to be effective. In fact, the more intense the odor, the less pleasant it becomes.

By blending together two or more pure essential oils, a synergy can be created that is more powerful than the individual oils. The interaction of the oils with one another gives an added vibrancy to the blend. Synergistic blends are achieved by combining oils that complement each other. For example, the calming effects of lavender and bergamot or rosemary work well together. Oils with opposite effects, such as a soothing oil and a stimulating oil should not be blended. It is also important that the blend has a pleasing scent. Table 9.4 presents a basic assortment of essential oils that can be blended to address most any complaint.

Table 9.4 An Aromatherapeutic Toolkit

Oil	Use
Basil	Decrease sinus congestion; soothe GI tract, aid digestion; decrease headache; decrease anxiety; decrease menstrual cramps
Bergamot	Decrease anxiety, decrease depression; urinary antiseptic; acne, disinfectant for wounds, abscesses, boils
Cedarwood	Decrease respiratory congestion and coughs, expectorant; for pain swelling of arthritis; antifungal for skin rashes
Chamomile	Soothe muscle aches, sprains, swollen joints; GI antispasmodic; rub on abdomen for colic, indigestion, gas; decrease anxiety, stress-related headaches; decrease insomnia; can be used with children
Clary sage	Induce sleep; increase sense of well-being; massage or warm compress for menstrual cramps; do not use in pregnancy until onset of labor
Coriander	Improve digestion, decrease colic, decrease diarrhea; decrease muscle aches and stiffness in joints; decrease mental fatigue and increase memory and mental function
Cypress	Massage or cold compress for rheumatic aches; bruising or varicose veins; respiratory antispasmodic (put couple of drops on hanky and inhale deeply), decrease coughs, asthma, bronchitis
Elemi	Boost immune system; cystitis; speed bone healing (massage in prior to casting); increase healing of cuts, sores, wounds; cool inflamed skin; sedative
Eucalyptus	Feels cool to skin and warm to muscles; decrease fever; relieve pain; anti-inflammatory; antiseptic, antiviral, and expectorant to respiratory system in steam inhalation; boost immune system
Frankincense	Bronchodilatory, acts on mucus enabling sputum to be expelled; infected sores; deepen breathing to induce calmness; incense creates a state conducive to prayer
Geranium	Antibacterial; insecticidal; antidepressant; improve yeast infections; first aid on minor cuts and burns
Ginger	Help ward off colds; calm upset stomach, decrease nausea; soothe sprains, muscle spasms
Green apple	Reduce headache severity; decrease anxiety; aid in weight reduction program; reduce symptoms of claustrophobia
Jasmine	Uplifting and stimulating, antidepressant; massage abdomen and lower back for menstrual cramps
Juniper	Calming, decrease stress; diuretic; muscle aches and pains
Lavender	Calming, sedative, for insomnia; massage around temples for headache; inhale to speed recovery from colds, flu; massage chest to decrease congestion; heal burns

Oil	Use
Lemon balm	Calming, sedative, decrease anxiety, decrease depression; antiseptic, antiviral, antifungal, eliminate cold sores
Lemon grass	Sedative; skin antiseptic for acne
Marjoram	Insomnia, decrease tension; muscle and joint pain; inhale to clear sinuses and clear congestion; massage abdomen for menstrual cramps
Neroli	Gentle sedative for insomnia, panic attacks; massage abdomen for irritable bowel syndrome
Orange	General tonic; decrease anxiety; GI antispasmodic for colic and indigestion; massage abdomen for constipation; can be used with children
Peppermint	Increase alertness; GI antispasmodic for colic and indigestion; massage on temples for headache; decongestant for colds, flu
Rose	Antidepressant; increase alertness; compress for eyestrain, headaches; use in massage for PMS
Rosemary	Stimulating; increase circulation to skin; compress on swollen joints; decrease respiratory congestion; antifungal, antibacterial; deodorize the air
Sandalwood	Calm and cool body; decrease inflammation; drops on handkerchief for sore throat, congestion; in bath water for cystitis; improve chapped dry skin; increase sense of peace in meditation or prayer
Tea Tree	First aid kit in a bottle; antifungal, good for athlete's foot; soothe insect bites, stings, cuts, wounds; in bath for yeast infection; drops on handkerchief for coughs, congestion
Vetiver	Stimulate production of red blood cells; increase circulation; induce restful sleep; decrease tension

Aromatherapy at Home

You can experiment with the use of aromatherapy in a number of ways. Essential oils can be combined with carrier oils and used for back rubs and foot rubs in helping clients relax and decrease their levels of anxiety. Essential oils can be diffused into the air to alter the structure of molecules creating unpleasant odors, thus refreshing the environment with more than just a pleasant smell. Diffusion of essential oils can also help boost your immune system, decrease anxiety and stress, aid restful sleep, and speed recovery.

SOOTHING POTIONS

ROSEWATER

Instead of using soap, try splashing your face with rosewater, a simple infusion from rose petals that contains some of the flowers' essential oils. Rose oil has mild antiseptic and anti-inflammatory properties, can constrict the tiny blood vessels in your skin to reduce redness, and it's also used in aromatherapy to calm your nerves and elevate your mood. You can buy rosewater in any natural food store, but you can also make your own. Put a handful of fresh rose petals into a small saucepan, add enough water to cover the petals completely, simmer for 15 minutes, then remove the pan from the heat. When it's completely cooled, strain away the petals and transfer your rosewater to a clean glass bottle.

CALENDULA SALVE

Calendula is a relative of the common marigold and is an easy-to-grow perennial. Calendula flowers have antibacterial and antifungal properties and also speed up the skin's healing process. The salve is extremely effective for diaper rash and other skin irritations. You can buy the salve, or you can make your own from home-grown or store-bought calendula flowers. Grind one-half cup of dried flowers in a blender or clean coffee grinder. Combine with one cup of olive oil in a glass canning jar with a lid. Place the jar in a large pan filled with enough water to cover the bottom half of the jar, and put the pan in the oven. Turn the oven on to the lowest temperature possible and allow the herbs to gently heat in the oil for several hours. Remove from the oven and allow to cool to room temperature. Filter the oil through a strainer lined with several layers of cheesecloth. To make the salve, place one-half cup of the herbal oil in a small heavy saucepan and add one-eighth cup of grated beeswax. Gently heat until the beeswax is completely melted. Test the consistency of the salve by placing a teaspoon of the mixture into the freezer for a minute. If you want a firmer salve, add more beeswax, and if you want a softer salve, add more oil. Pour the salve into small wide-mouth glass jars with lids. If stored in a cool, dark place, the salve will stay fresh for about one year.

As a general rule, you should purchase essential oils in natural and health food stores rather than stores selling beauty products and perfumes. They should be stored in dark vials, tightly closed and away from heat, light, or dampness. Professional aromatherapists use up to 300 oils. Most people can meet their home needs with fewer than 30 or even just 10: chamomile, clove, eucalyptus, geranium, lavender, lemon, peppermint, rosemary, tea tree, and thyme.

THE ABSOLUTE MINIMUM

- Aromatherapy uses essential oils from all sorts of plants to trigger specific physiological reactions in the skin and the olfactory system.

- Aromatherapy has been used for millennia; ancient Egyptians used many of the same oils and balms used by aromatherapists today.

- You can experiment with aromatherapy at home using a small selection of oils that can be blended to provide energy, ease tension, and increase the sensory pleasure of your home.

RESOURCES

- Institute of Aromatherapy

  www.aromatherapy4u.com

- National Association for Holistic Aromatherapy (NAHA)

  www.naha.org

- Smell and Taste Treatment and Research Foundation

  www.smellandtaste.org

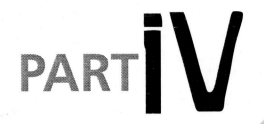

PART IV

MANUAL HEALING PRACTICES

10

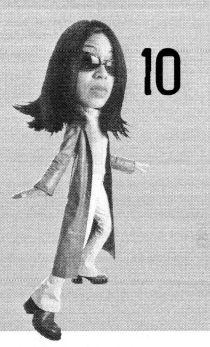

CHIROPRACTIC PRACTICE

The word chiropractic comes from two Greek words *cheir* (hand) and *praktikos* (practical), which were combined to mean "done by hand." Chiropractic, by numbers of practitioners, is the third largest independent health profession in the United States, following conventional medicine and dentistry. Chiropractors are primary health care providers, licensed both for diagnosis and treatment. The practice is limited by procedure (manipulation of the spine) and excludes surgery and prescription medications.

What Is Chiropractic?

Manipulation, as a healing technique, was practiced long before chiropractic. Chinese artifacts, as early as 2700 BC, describe manipulation of the spine. In 1500 BC, the Greeks gave written instructions on how to manipulate the lumbar spine for back care. Hippocrates used spinal manipulation to reposition vertebrae and cure a variety of dysfunctions. Galen, a Greek physician, anatomist, and physiologist, born over two hundred years after Hippocrates, also used manipulation and reported the cure of a patient's hand weakness and numbness through manipulation of the seventh cervical vertebra. Hippocrates and Galen helped form the foundation of Renaissance medicine, during which manipulative healers were known as "bone-setters." The "father of surgery," Ambroise Pare, born about 1517, incorporated manipulation into his treatment of patients. In the centuries that followed, manipulative techniques were passed down from generation to generation, often within families.

Chiropractic was founded in 1895 by Daniel David Palmer, a self-educated American healer. Palmer administered the first chiropractic adjustment to Harvey Lillard, a janitor who had gone deaf 17 years earlier while stooping in a mine. Palmer found what he called a misaligned vertebra, which he manipulated, allowing Lillard to stand up straight, free of back pain, and with his hearing restored. Within two years of this discovery, Palmer founded his Chiropractic School and Cure while at the same time developing the underlying concepts. In 1906, a split in the profession occurred that still exists today. Several faculty members, including John Howard, left Palmer College because of significant differences with Palmer's son, B. J. Palmer. B. J. believed that spinal *subluxation* or misalignment of the spinal vertebrae, was the cause of all disease whereas Howard believed that additional causes were generally present. Howard opened his National School of Chiropractic around a broad-based and scientific educational curriculum. To this day, those who follow Palmer's path are called "straight" chiropractors, while those who follow the Howard model are called "mixer" chiropractors.

Chiropractors are licensed in all states of the United States as well as in many other countries. The 16 American chiropractic colleges graduate more than 2,800 chiropractors each year. Colleges also exist in Canada, Australia, England, France, and Japan. Chiropractic education requires at least 60 undergraduate credit hours, including many in the basic sciences. Chiropractic college is a five-year program including courses in anatomy, physiology, pathology, and diagnosis, as well as spinal adjusting, nutrition, physical therapy, and rehabilitation. Educational standards in the United States are supervised by a government-recognized accrediting agency, the Council of Chiropractic Education.

Chiropractors function almost entirely in free-standing private practice. Some continue their education with postdoctoral training in specialty areas such as radiology, orthopedics, neurology, behavioral medicine, family practice, occupational health, and sports medicine.

How Does Chiropractic Work?

The assumption underlying all chiropractic treatment is that spinal misalignment impairs the transmission of information—nerve impulses—through the spinal cord, causing pain and disruptions throughout the central nervous system and the entire body.

Anatomy

The adult spinal column is comprised of 26 vertebrae: 7 cervical (in the neck), 12 thoracic (upper back), 5 lumbar (lower back), 1 sacral (at the hips), and 1 coccygeal (at the tailbone). These vertebrae provide attachment for various muscles and protection for the spinal cord; they are separated by intervertebral disks. Several curves in the vertebral column increase its strength. The spinal cord, housed in the vertebral canal, conducts sensory and motor impulses to and from the brain and controls many reflexes. It connects to the rest of the body through the 31 pairs of spinal nerves originating from the cord.

The vertebrae, with the exception of the first and second cervical, are much alike and are composed of a body, an arch, and seven projections called processes. See Figure 10.1. Vertebrae are connected at the processes by a cartilaginous structure called a facet joint, which is encased in a strong, fibrous joint capsule that prevents the joint from coming apart. The structure and health of these connections are the primary concern of chiropractic. The other anatomical feature that is of concern to chiropractic is the sacroiliac joint, which is formed where the sacrum attaches to the ilia.

Foundations of Chiropractic Treatment

Chiropractic believes that the body possesses a unique internal wisdom that continually strives to maintain a state of health within the body. This body wisdom means that every person has an innate healing potential. Accessing this internal healing system is the goal of the healing arts. In addition, it is believed that a balanced, natural diet and regular exercise are essential to proper bodily function and good health. The assumptions of chiropractic are as follows:

FIGURE 10.1

The bones in your backbone: Structure of the spinal vertebrae.

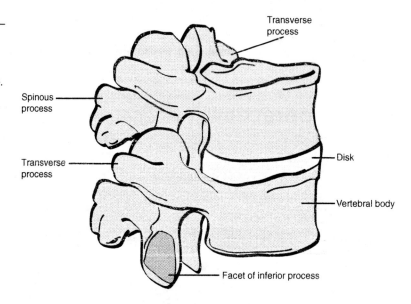

Transverse process

Spinous process

Transverse process

Disk

Vertebral body

Facet of inferior process

- Structure and function exist in intimate relation with one another.
- Structural distortions can cause functional abnormalities.
- The vertebral subluxation (misalignment) is a significant form of structural distortion and leads to a variety of functional abnormalities.
- The nervous system plays a prominent role in the restoration and maintenance of proper bodily function.
- Subluxation influences bodily function primarily through neurologic means.
- Chiropractic adjustment is a specific and definitive method for the correction of vertebral subluxation.

Chiropractic addresses the application of this knowledge to diagnose and treat structural dysfunctions that affect the nervous system. Since the nervous system is highly developed in humans, it influences all other systems in the body, thereby playing a significant role in health and disease.

The Limits of Misalignment

Chiropractic believes that health is a state of balance, especially of the nervous and musculoskeletal systems. When the spine is fully aligned, nerve energy flows freely to every cell and organ in the body. This free flow of energy nurtures the innate ability of the body to work effectively and coordinate normal body functions.

Traditionally, chiropractic viewed illness and disease as caused by misalignment of the spinal vertebrae, referred to as vertebral subluxation, leading to irritation and dysfunction of nerves and blood vessels. The disrupted flow of impulses was thought to interfere with normal muscle function, respiration, heartbeat, arterial tone, digestion, and resistance to disease. A more recent theory is that of intervertebral motion dysfunction. This motion theory contends that loss of mobility in the facet joints, rather than misalignment, is the key factor in the concept of subluxation. Subluxation can be caused by just about anything—falls, injuries, genetic spinal weaknesses, improper sleeping habits, poor posture, obesity, stress, and occupational hazards.

Although this "one cause" philosophy has been a central concept in chiropractic history, few chiropractors today would endorse this simplistic formulation of illness. They recognize the existence of bacteria and viruses in creating disease, especially in a susceptible person. Susceptibility depends on many factors, one of which is spinal misalignment. Although it now embraces a multifaceted explanation of disease, the chiropractic treatment of choice is spinal adjustment.

About Chiropractic Treatment

Ninety percent of those seeking chiropractic have neuromusculoskeletal symptoms or disorders, primarily back pain, neck pain, and headaches. The central focus of chiropractic diagnosis is the determination of when and where spinal manual therapy (SMT) is appropriate. The diagnostic process also determines what type of adjustment would be most appropriate. Unlike conventional medicine, which typically assumes that the site of a pain is the site of its cause, chiropractors evaluate the site of pain in a regional and whole-body context. Joint pain in the upper extremities, for example, can be caused by injury or pathology in the joint but may also originate from cervical spine dysfunction. Similarly, the source of joint pain in the lower extremities can be in the lumbar spine. The chiropractic assumption is that the source of the pain should be sought along the path of the nerves leading to and from the site of the symptoms. This whole-body approach is a hallmark of chiropractic.

The Chiropractic Assessment

A detailed history is the first step in chiropractic diagnosis. The chiropractor asks about the pattern and quality of the pain and its chronology. Is the pain constant or intermittent? Is the pain a dull ache, a nagging sensation, or a burning sensation? What causes the pain to get worse? What causes the pain to get better? The answers to these types of questions are key to the diagnostic process.

The chiropractic physician consistently assesses a number of back pain risk factors that are critical to diagnosis. Individual factors contributing to back pain include older age, tallness, obesity, smoking, decreased muscle strength, decreased flexibility, lack of physical conditioning, and multiple pregnancies. Other health conditions are considered, such as osteoporosis, multiple myeloma, osteoarthritis, scoliosis, and ruptured disc. Psychological factors include the person's levels of anxiety, stress, and pain tolerance. Occupational risk factors for back pain include heavy physical work; frequent bending, twisting, lifting, pushing, pulling; repetitive strain; and injury or accidents. Recreational risk factors include hockey, football, gymnastics, golf, racquetball, bowling, squash, handball, tennis, backpacking, wrestling, skiing, and other high-impact sports. All applicable risk factors are noted during the history.

Relying heavily on hands-on procedures, the chiropractic physician uses palpation to determine both structural and functional problems. These hands-on procedures are complemented by a neurological physical examination, testing nerve function, reflexes, coordination and muscle function. It is the same neurological assessment done by a conventional physician.

Following the neurological evaluation is the motion palpation exam in which the chiropractor physically examines the spine, noting how it feels, as well as how the client says it feels. The client is gently moved into and out of various postures during this part of the exam. Some postures are done standing while others are done while lying down. This process often informs the chiropractor what movements or positions reproduce or aggravate the pain. X-rays to confirm diagnostic findings may or may not be done.

Hypermobility of spinal joints is diagnosed by the sound of a repeated click when a joint is moved through its normal range of motion. This unstable type of subluxation is related to flaccid ligaments and is more problematic than the fixated type of subluxation. Hypermobile joints should not be forcibly manipulated since manipulation can move the joint beyond the safe range of motion and increase the degree of hypermobility. Rather, nearby joints that have become immobile to compensate for the unstable joint can be manipulated, and muscle strength and tone can be increased with exercise.

The chiropractor rules out pathologies that are contraindicative to spinal manual therapy (SMT). For example, advanced, degenerative joint disease would rule out all forms of SMT that use significant force on the joint. Chiropractic treatment is not appropriate in the case of spinal infections, fractures, or tumors, which fortunately are fairly rare. In addition, SMT is not done on a woman in late pregnancy or on people whose pain is increased with manipulation. Diagnosis determines appropriate chiropractic treatment, referral for appropriate conventional medical care, or concurrent care.

The Chiropractic Cure

Three primary clinical goals guide chiropractic intervention:

- The first goal is to reduce or eliminate people's pain. Typically this goal is the client's primary, and often only goal.

- The second clinical goal is to correct the subluxation, thereby restoring bio-mechanical balance to reestablish shock absorption, leverage, and range of motion. In addition, muscles and ligaments are strengthened by spinal rehabilitative exercises to increase resistance to further injury.

- The third clinical goal is preventative maintenance to assure the problem does not recur. This goal is comparable to the idea of having teeth cleaned periodically to prevent decay. Maintenance intervals vary from person to person depending on lifestyle.

Back pain is a leading cause of disability and the second most common reason (after the common cold) people visit a doctor. Chiropractors have two times the number of visits for back pain as conventional physicians. Most chiropractors also treat peripheral joints—elbows, knees, and shoulders. In 1994, a panel for the Agency for Health Care Policy and Research of the United States Department of Health and Human Services concluded that spinal manual therapy speeds recovery from acute low back pain and recommended it either in combination with or as a replacement for nonsteroid, anti-inflammatory drugs. At the same time the panel rejected many methods used for years by conventional medicine such as bed rest, traction, and various other physical therapy modalities and cautioned against spinal surgery except in the most severe cases.

Chiropractors manipulate their clients' spines by using their hands to apply pressure in specific locations and directions. The skill lies in the ability to be specific about which joint is being manipulated, which is especially important in the presence of any unstable joints. A chiropractor has 10–20 different ways of manipulating every movable joint in the body. Chiropractors also practice soft-tissue manipulation to stretch contracted muscles and decrease muscle spasms.

High-velocity, low-amplitude (HVLA) thrust adjustment is the most common form of manipulation. It is performed by manually moving a joint to the end-point of its normal range of motion, isolating it by local pressure on bony prominences, and then giving a swift, specific, low-amplitude thrust.

Often a series of these thrusts are applied to the back and neck. When the facet joints are forced apart, a small vacuum is created and then released, which creates a popping sound much like when people crack their knuckles. This manipulation does not cause pain, though people may feel a little discomfort the next day due to rebalancing of the contracted muscles. This sensation can be compared to muscular soreness at the beginning of a weight-training program. Other adjusting methods include low-velocity thrust adjustment with mechanically assisted drop-piece tables, various light-touch techniques, ultrasound, and electrical muscle stimulation.

ENERGY BOOSTER
Poor posture robs your body of energy. You may spend many hours of your day walking incorrectly or slumped in a chair, which interrupts the flow of energy and oxygen through your body and spinal cord. Take a moment to sit up or stand straight. Imagine that a cord is attached to the top of your head, pulling it gently toward the sky. This image helps readjust your posture. Feel your head, neck, shoulders, and spine relax as they realign from a constricting position. This imagery, practiced either sitting or standing, will revive you.

More Than Just Back-Cracking

As holistic practitioners, chiropractors work with many facets of their clients' lifestyles. Nutrition education is provided, exercise programs are designed, rehabilitation measures are planned, correct posture and lifting techniques are explained, and activities of daily living are assessed and improved. Conditions commonly seen by a chiropractor include the following:

- Lower back syndromes
- Mid back conditions
- Neck syndromes
- Headaches
- Carpal tunnel syndrome
- Sciatica
- Muscle spasms
- Sports-related injuries
- Whiplash and accident-related injuries
- Arthritic conditions
- Shoulder conditions
- Torticolis
- Extremity trauma

THE ABSOLUTE MINIMUM

- Chiropractic practitioners address their patients' health concerns by locating, correcting, and preventing spinal misalignment, which is believed to adversely effect the nervous system and overall health.

- Chiropractic education is a serious, multi-year undertaking, and chiropractors, the third-largest group of independent health professionals in the U.S., are licensed in every state.

- Chiropractic treatment consists of both direct spinal manipulation to correct misalignments and education and strength building practices to prevent further misalignment.

RESOURCES

- American Chiropractic Association

   www.amerchiro.org

- Palmer Chiropractic University

   www.palmer.edu

- National University of Health Sciences

   www.nuhs.edu

- Federation of Chiropractic Licensing Boards

   www.fclb.org

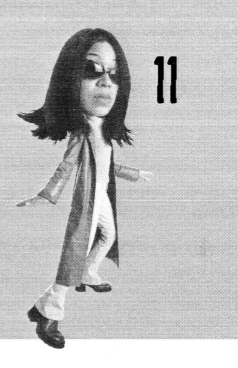

11

Massage

Massage therapy, the scientific manipulation of the soft tissues of the body, is a healing art, an act of physical caring, and a way of communicating without words. The goal of massage therapy is to achieve or increase health and well-being and to help the body heal itself. Although massage therapists may hold general views of health and well-being, massage therapy has no specific theoretical framework or diagnostic system of disease.

What Is Massage?

The idea that touch can heal is an old one. Cave paintings in the Pyrenees show that 15,000 years ago people treated injuries with what looks like massage. References to massage are found in 4,000-year-old Chinese medical texts. Hippocrates wrote, "The physician must be acquainted with many things and assuredly with rubbing" (the ancient Greek and Roman term for massage). Some of the greatest physicians in history advocated massage, including Celsus (25 BC–50 AD), Galen (131–200), and Avicenna (980–1037). Ambroise Pare (1517–1590) the "father of surgery," William Harvey (1578–1657), who demonstrated the circulation of blood, and Herman Boerhaave (1668–1738), who introduced the clinical method of teaching medicine, all utilized massage as a healing technique. Roman gladiators were massaged before entering the arenas and eighteenth century Swedish cavalrymen were rubbed down between battles. In the Middle Ages, Christians viewed massage as the work of the devil and many therapists were burned at the stake as witches. Remnants of this attitude have continued into the twentieth century as massage is sometimes assumed to be a front for prostitution.

The German emperor Frederick II (thirteenth century) was curious to know what language children would speak if they were raised without hearing any words at all. Stealing a number of newborns from their parents, he gave them to nurses who physically cared for the infants but were forbidden to cuddle or talk to them. All the children died before they could talk. This discovery was important: Tactile stimulation can be a matter of life and death. (Cosmic justice came to Frederick in 1250, when he suffered a wrenching bout of dysentery and died.)

Infant massage dates to ancient times. An Indian medical text from 1800 BC recommends diet, exercise, and massage as healing techniques. The practice spread to the United States in the 1980s after the publication of *Infant Massage* by Vimala Schneider McClure, and *Baby Massage* by Amelia Auckett. Both women received their massage training in India.

In many areas of the world, massage serves as an integral part of health systems. In the former Soviet Union, Germany, China, and Japan, massage therapists work along with physicians in the hospital setting as important members of the health care team. In Germany today, doctors will write a prescription for 10 massage treatments as readily as for a bottle of tranquilizers, and massage is covered by Germany's national health insurance plan.

Massage in the United States

Massage was introduced to Americans in the early nineteenth century by two New York physicians who were trained in Sweden. The first massage therapy clinics were opened by Swedish physicians after the Civil War and had among their clients members of congress and Presidents Harrison and Grant. At first, physicians performed massage, but they eventually delegated the technique to nurses and physical therapists and by the mid-twentieth century, massage therapy was virtually abandoned by most health care professionals except nurses. Advanced medical technology, sophisticated equipment, and nurses assuming more of a management role have left little time for hands-on nursing care. An upsurge of interest in the field began in the 1970s with Dr. Dolores Kreiger and Dr. Martha Rogers, two nurse pioneers who advocated the art and caring form of touch in nursing practice. At the turn of the new century, nurses are returning to their tradition in providing comfort and care through the use of touch and massage.

Compared with members of other cultures, people in the United States are generally touch-phobic and touch-deprived. Cross-cultural studies have revealed that people in the United States have one of the lowest rates of casual touch in the world. When psychologist Sidney Jourard observed rates of casual touch among couples in cafes, he reported the highest rates in Puerto Rico (180 times per hour) and Paris (110 times per hour), and one of the lowest in the United States (two times per hour). French parents and children touch each other three times more frequently than their U.S. counterparts. French teens demonstrate significantly more casual touching of friends than U.S. adolescents, who are more likely to fiddle with their rings, crack their knuckles, and demonstrate other forms of self-stimulation. Other studies have found cultures that are more physically affectionate toward infants and children tend to have lower rates of adult violence. In spite of advertising pleas to "reach out and touch someone," the majority of North Americans have precious little physical contact with family members, friends, and co-workers.

Concerns have been escalating about "inappropriate" touch, sexual abuse, and sexual harassment in schools and workplaces in the United States. Some schools have instituted "teach, but don't touch" policies. It is rare to see teachers put their hands on the shoulder of a child who is crying. Sadly, to protect themselves from being accused of inappropriate touch, many people are not touching at all. While concern for protecting children from those who would touch inappropriately is valid, the implications of a "hands-off" barrier have significant negative effects on growth, development, and emotional well-being.

Perhaps in response to this trend, massage, a hands-on touch therapy, has reached out to an ever-widening U.S. audience. Massage is now the third most common form of alternative treatment in the United States, after relaxation techniques and chiropractic. The power of touch has people in the United States spending almost $4 billion yearly on professional massages as 25 million individuals make 60 million visits each year. These numbers do not include institutions that offer massage in the workplace or the children of thousands of parents who learn baby massage.

Twenty-five states, the District of Columbia, and some cities require massage thera-pists to have 500 or more hours of education from a recognized school and some states also require the passing of a licensing exam. The curriculum consists of 300 hours of massage theory and technique, 100 hours of anatomy and physiology, and 100 hours of additional courses to meet the school's specific program objectives. Additional states are expected to adopt licensing acts in the near future. The American Massage Therapy Association accredits 60 programs throughout the United States. Curriculums must consist of 500 or more hours and include specified hours of anatomy, physiology, massage theory and practice, and ethics. The National Certification Exam was first administered in 1992, and by 1997, 27,000 therapists were certified. The International Association of Infant Massage certifies instructors who take four days of training, read course material, and pass a take-home exam.

How Does Massage Work?

Touch is the fundamental medium of massage therapy. It is, however, more than just mechanical manipulation. Touch is a form of communication, thus one of the most significant benefits is the comfort of human care conveyed by the therapist. Massage communicates gentleness and connection, trust and receiving, and peace and alertness.

Massage helps the body to heal itself and is aimed at achieving or increasing health and well-being. Only now is science beginning to catch up with people when it comes to appreciating the importance—and the power—of touch.

The stronger, sustained touch used in massage can have an even greater effect than other forms of touch. A skilled massage therapist not only stretches and loosens muscle and connective tissue, but also greatly improves blood flow and the move-ment of lymph fluid throughout the body. Massage speeds the removal of metabolic waste products resulting from exercise or inactivity, allowing more oxygen and nutrients to reach the cells and tissues. The release of muscular tension also helps to unblock and balance the overall flow of life energy throughout the body known as *qi, prana,* or subtle energy. In addition, massage can stimulate the release of endor-phins and serotonin in the brain and nervous system.

Skin: The Organ You're In

In many ways, human beings are wired for touch. The skin is the body's largest organ, covering almost 20 square feet and accounting for nearly one-quarter of the body's total weight. As many as five million touch receptors in the skin—3,000 in a fingertip—send messages via the spinal cord to the brain. The sense of touch is the earliest to develop in the human embryo and at less than eight weeks of gestation, a light stroking of the face will cause bending of the neck and trunk away from the source of stimulation. The skin has four main functions: protection from mechanical and radiation injuries, and from invasion by foreign substances; as a sense organ; as a temperature regulator; and as a metabolic organ. Of all the sensory organs, the skin is the most important. People can survive without the senses of sight, sound, smell, and taste, but would find it difficult to survive without the functions performed by the skin.

Touch

Touch is a primal need, as necessary for growth and development as food, clothing, or shelter. Touch can be thought of as a nutrient transmitted through the skin in many different ways: holding, cuddling, nuzzling, caressing, and massage. From the bonding of parent and newborn to the holding the hand of a dying loved one, touch is the most intimate and powerful form of communication between people. It can be aggressive as in the spanking of a child or a punch in the face. It can be tender as in the hug that comforts a crying friend or the touch of a lover. Even casual touch has an effect. Waitresses who touched their customers on the hand or shoulder as they returned change, for example, received larger tips than those who did not. Politicians act on this knowledge when they reach out to touch potential voters.

Trigger Points: A Pain in the Neck

When a person is injured or bodily systems are malfunctioning, trigger points or pain reflexes appear throughout the body. A trigger point is a "knot" of tensed muscles, which, when stimulated, triggers a referred pain response in other parts of the body. Some of the trigger points are in the area of the injury or problem, while others are at a distance. Rubbing and exerting pressure on these points have been found to have a positive effect on the healing process.

Fascia and Fascial Restrictions

The *fascia* is the tough connective tissue that exists in the body almost like a three-dimensional web from head to foot. If somehow every structure of the body were removed except the fascia, the body would retain its shape. Every muscle, bone, organ, nerve, and blood vessel of the body is covered with fascia like a continuous cellophane wrapping. It varies in thickness and density and in the amount of collagenous fiber, elastic fiber, and tissue fluid it contains. The function of the fascia is to support cells, muscles, groups of muscles and organs and to act as a shock absorber. At the cellular level, fascia creates the interstitial spaces and is important in cellular respiration, elimination, metabolism, fluid, and lymphatic flow.

Each time a person experiences a trauma, undergoes an inflammatory process, or suffers from poor posture over time, the fascial system becomes restricted and the person loses flexibility and spontaneity of motion. As the fascia continue to slowly tighten, an abnormal pressure develops on the nerves, muscles, bones, or organs, resulting in poor cellular efficiency, necrosis, pain, and dysfunction throughout the body.

THE BENEFITS OF MASSAGE

PHYSICAL LEVEL
- Relieves muscle tension and stiffness
- Reduces muscle spasm and tension
- Speeds recovery from exertion
- Improves joint flexibility and range of motion
- Increases ease and efficiency of movement
- Improves posture
- Stimulates lymphatic circulation, which decreases edema
- Improves local circulation, which increases healing of injured tissues
- Lowers blood pressure, slows heart rate
- Eases tension headaches

MENTAL LEVEL
- Induces a relaxed state of alertness
- Reduces mental stress thus clearing the mind
- Increases capacity for clearer thinking

EMOTIONAL LEVEL
- Satisfies the need for caring and nurturing touch
- Increases feelings of well-being, decreases mild depression
- Enhances self-image
- Reduces levels of anxiety
- Increases awareness of mind-body connection

What Are the Different Types of Massage?

The first massage therapy appointment usually begins with questions about one's physical condition, medical history, and current aches and pains. The therapist determines what a client hopes to gain from the massage. The client undresses in private and uses a sheet or blanket for draping. The individual decides whether underwear is on or off. The client lies on a cushioned table and the therapist uncovers only that part of the body being massaged, using oil or lotion to help the hands move smoothly. It is recommended that clients not eat just before a massage and drink extra water afterward to clear the body of toxins released from deep tissues. At home, clients are encouraged to enjoy a salt bath as another aid in detoxifying the body. Add one-half cup each of sea salt, Epsom salt, and baking soda to a tub of warm water for the salt bath.

From hour-long massages in therapists' offices to 10-minute massages at the workplace, a massage is available for practically every body and budget. Massage therapists offer their services in a wide variety of settings such as private practice clinics, health clubs and fitness centers, chiropractic offices, nursing homes and hospitals, salons and resorts, on-site in the workplace, and even in clients' homes. There are almost as many styles of massage as there are practitioners. Most therapists combine a variety of methods in their work, which allows them to tailor each session to the specific needs of the client.

caution

Massage should not be used for some situations:

- Phlebitis/thrombosis
- Severe varicose veins
- Any acute inflammation of the skin, soft tissue, or joints
- Areas of hemorrhage or heavy tissue damage
- Unregulated blood pressure
- Febrile state
- Herniated disc
- Recent fractures or sprains
- Some types of cancer

Swedish Massage

Peter Ling of Sweden developed Swedish massage about 150 years ago. He integrated ancient Asian massage with a Western understanding of anatomy and physiology. It is the most common form of massage in the United States. Swedish massage uses a system of long gliding strokes, as well as kneading and friction techniques on the more superficial layers of the muscles, combined with active and passive movements of the joints. It is used primarily for a full-body massage to promote general relaxation, improve circulation and range of motion, and relieve muscle tension.

Swedish massage uses five basic strokes. *Effleurage,* French for "touching," is the introductory stroke. The therapist uses the whole hand providing long, gliding strokes relaxing the central nervous system and preparing the local area for the other strokes. *Petrissage* involves grasping muscle groups and lifting them, stretching them away from the bones and then kneading or rolling them. This technique is the closest in imitating exercise because it makes the muscles contract. This stroke is used mostly on flaccid muscles that need to have their contractile ability increased. Petrissage also stimulates the central nervous system and therefore is not used with clients who have cerebral vascular dysfunctions. *Friction* involves using the fingers and thumbs to press on small areas and move in a circular motion around the area. *Vibration* involves placing the hands on a muscle group and moving them back and forth quickly in a shaking motion. *Tapotement* involves striking the skin with the outside edges of the hands, fingers, or cupped palms to stimulate circulation.

Shiatsu Massage

In Japanese, *shi* means "finger" and *atsu* means "pressure." Shiatsu massage is the Japanese adaptation of acupressure. Like Chinese acupuncture and acupressure, shiatsu is based on the idea that life energy, *chi*, flows along invisible pathways called meridians. Health is related to a free flow of energy, and illness is caused by blockages to the flow. Blocked energy can cause physical discomforts, so the aim is to release the blocks associated with the discomfort or disease and rebalance the energy flow. Therapists use their hands, elbows, and even their feet to press for about 30 seconds on each point. Depending on the way it is done, Shiatsu can be gentle or quite forceful. Done on a floor mat rather than a massage table, a typical Shiatsu session lasts about an hour.

Trigger Point Massage

Trigger point massage is a type of deep massage, in which the fingers are used to release knots and tender spots in muscles. Rubbing and exerting pressure on these points has been found to have a positive effect on the healing process by interrupting the cycle of spasm and pain. Techniques are similar to those used in shiatsu but are based on Western anatomy and physiology. Trigger point massage is typically a technique incorporated into Swedish or sports massage.

Sports Massage

Sports massage uses techniques of Swedish massage and Shiatsu massage but focuses on parts of the body that are likely to be stressed by a particular sport. It takes less time than Swedish or Shiatsu and is usually more vigorous. For example, runners might need to have their hamstrings worked extensively. This technique also concentrates on reducing or eliminating factors that interfere with human performance such as muscle spasms, tendonitis, and muscle fatigue.

Prior to the athletic event, massage loosens, warms, and readies the muscle for intensive use, especially when combined with stretching. Besides helping prevent injury, it can improve performance and endurance. Post-event massage relieves pain, prevents stiffness, and returns the muscles to their normal state more rapidly. The use of massage in sports health care is increasing rapidly in both training and competition. Recreational athletes also have discovered the benefits of sports massage as a regular part of their workouts.

Rolfing

Developed by the late biochemist Ida P. Rolf, *Rolfing* (also known as structural integration) is a system of whole-body manipulation in which the rolfer uses the fingers, knuckles, and elbows to stretch the fascia, which tends to bind up because of injury, bad posture, emotional problems, or genetic weaknesses. The fascia is stretched to release patterns of tension and rigidity and return the body to a state of correct alignment. Other massage therapists work by applying smooth strokes over muscles; rolfers press deeply into muscle tissue and fascia to release them. Clients are asked to breathe deeply during the session and visualize the muscle lengthening. The new Rolfing method is gentler and far less painful than the original style of treatment. Practitioners use a broad range of touch and pressure from feather-light to deep massage. When performed with the right sensitivity, even deep and heavy pressure may not be painful.

Executive Massage

Executive massage is done with the client fully dressed, seated on a portable massage chair. The face is supported by a doughnut-shaped pillow, which allows for easy breathing. The sessions, which last 10–20 minutes, involve massage of the head, neck, back, arms, and hands. This type of massage is often provided in the workplace or in shopping malls. The purpose of the massage is to decrease tension, reduce stress, and enhance people's adaptive capabilities.

Thai Massage

Some people call Thai massage passive yoga, as the receiver is fully clothed, lies on a futon, and is deeply stretched, compressed, and gently rocked. The whole body of the therapist is used to treat the whole body of the receiver. The experience feels like a combination of yoga, shiatsu, and meditation. Point pressure and kneading of the tissues is similar to massage techniques. Yoga techniques used in Thai massage involve positioning the client in numerous stretches similar to yoga poses, then gently rocking the person to deepen the stretch and open the joints. The gentle rocking creates an energy flow through the different stretches. Thai massage gives the person the flexibility, inner organ massage, oxygenation of the blood, and quieting of the mind that comes with yoga, but because the receiver is passive the session becomes meditative. Sometimes the therapist stands on the recipient and gently rolls one foot on and off the body. This compression can be gentle to deep and can energize or relax the recipient.

Infant Massage

Infant massage is gaining in popularity in the United States. Researchers have found infant massage produces weight gains in premature infants, reduces complications in cocaine babies, and helps depressed mothers soothe their babies. In healthy babies it improves parent-infant bonding, eases painful procedures such as inoculations, reduces pain from teething and constipation, reduces colic, induces sleep, and makes parents feel good.

Self-Massage

Self-massage is a wonderful way for people to better acquaint themselves with their entire bodies. It is a process in which they learn to be aware of and release tensions and inhibitions, to reclaim parts of themselves that have been neglected, and to accept themselves as they are. Getting to know and appreciate one's body through touch is an important part of self-acceptance. The more in touch people are with themselves, the more they come in touch with the reality and experience of the world around them. Heightened awareness of the unity of body, mind, and spirit often leads to an increased perception of the unity of all nature. As it builds self-confidence and self-acceptance, this awareness enables people to respond with more compassion and caring to others.

Self-massage is done in a warm, comfortable, and quiet environment. Breath work and relaxation techniques are utilized to ground and center before the experience. Self-massage often begins with gazing at oneself naked in a mirror withholding judgment and criticism. Then the person finds a position that is relaxing and comfortable. Without a set route or sequence, individual senses guide self-massage. At times the whole body may be explored and massaged and at other times people may feel like spending the time on one part, such as the face and head. Self-massage is done slowly and rhythmically with the eyes closed so that all one's attention can be focused on the sensation.

Trying Massage at Home

One needs little more wisdom than that evinced by King Frederick to realize that massage is among the most accessible of alternative therapies. Alone or with a partner, massage can make a long day seem shorter and also yield real physiological benefits.

Mini-Massage (1–2 minutes)

Use the refined sesame oil sold in health food stores, not the heavy Chinese sesame oil. If you wish, you may use olive oil instead. Warm a quarter cup of oil in the microwave for 10–15 seconds, being careful not to overheat it.

Use one tablespoon of warm oil and rub it into your scalp. Use small, circular motions with the flat of your hand. Using your palm, massage the forehead from side to side and gently massage your temples using circular motions. Gently rub the outside of the ears. Massage both the front and the back of the neck.

Use a second tablespoon of warm oil and massage both feet using the flat of the hand. Massage each toe with your fingertips. Vigorously massage the soles of your feet. Sit quietly for a few seconds to relax and then shower or bathe as usual.

Full Body Massage (5–10 minutes)

Massage the scalp, ears, and neck with one tablespoon of warm oil as described above.

Using more oil, vigorously massage your arms using long strokes on the long parts and circular motions at the joints.

Adding oil as necessary, massage the chest, stomach, and lower abdomen using gentle circular strokes in a clockwise direction. Massage as much of your back and spine as you can reach.

Massage the legs as you did the arms using vigorous movements

With the remaining bit of oil, massage the feet as described above. Bathe with warm water and mild soap.

Partner Massage

- Set the mood with scented candles and soft music in a dimly lit room.
- Lay folded quilts on the floor rather than using your bed so you can easily move around your partner.
- Remove jewelry to avoid catching hairs as you work.

- Comfort your partner by covering her/him with a sheet and placing a pillow under the knees when lying on the back and under the ankles when lying on the front.
- Massage works best when strokes are lubricated. Any vegetable oil will work, but scented massage oils can add to the sense of relaxation and sensuality.
- Begin with both of you doing slow deep breathing to center and ground.
- Warm the oil by rubbing it between your hands before applying it.
- Begin with light strokes and proceed to deeper pressure only after the muscles in the area have relaxed and warmed up.
- Your partner should tell you if any strokes feel uncomfortable: too light, too deep, or on a tender spot.
- Take your time: ideally 2–3 minutes per foot, 10 minutes per leg, 15–20 minutes for the back, and 15 minutes for the front including 5 minutes on the face.
- Stroke toward the heart, instead of against the flow of blood returning to the heart.
- Never press directly on the spinal column, just on the muscles

Massage During Pregnancy

Childbirth nurses and nurse midwives have long advocated massage during pregnancy. A light, natural oil such as tangerine, almond, or safflower is used, avoiding the addition of any essential oils, which may have ill effects on the fetus. The benefits of massage during pregnancy are

- Relaxing. Massage helps reduce tension in the neck and shoulders and, in the later stages of pregnancy, in the lower back.
- Uplifting. Massage minimizes fatigue and improves the flow of energy and induces a general feeling of well-being.
- Improves circulation. Massage may help prevent varicose veins that may accompany pregnancy.
- Stimulates lymphatic drainage. Massage helps reduce fluid retention in the ankles and feet that often occurs during the later stages of pregnancy.
- Tones muscles. Massage helps relieve the pain of distended ligaments and decrease the tendency to cramp that may occur toward the fifth month of pregnancy.
- Maintains skin tone. Massage increases the skin's suppleness and elasticity and may help prevent stretch marks.

Infant Massage

Whether you are massaging a newborn or teaching parents infant massage, the process lasts for as little as a few minutes or as long as a half hour but should be performed only when a baby is willing. If a baby is crying, hiccupping, turning his head to the side, the massage should be discontinued and tried another time. The oil for infant massage should be a light-textured, unscented oil such as almond, coconut, or safflower oil. Infants should not be massaged with synthetic, petroleum-based products because they have no nutritional value and are not absorbed into the skin. The following are some gentle massage strokes for infants:

- Foot: press all over the bottom of the foot using the thumbs
- Leg: hold the leg like a baseball bat and move the hands up the leg squeezing slightly and turning in opposite directions
- Stomach: make scooping strokes, one hand following the other
- Chest: begin with both hands at the center and gently push out to the sides along the rib cage
- Back: with fingers spread apart, "comb" the back from the neck to the buttocks
- Hand: roll each finger between one's finger and thumb; press gently all over the palm, using the thumbs
- Face: make small circles around the jaw using the fingertips

THE ABSOLUTE MINIMUM

- Massage therapy combines the benefits of muscle manipulation, fascia relaxation, and another human's touch.
- Different types of massage may different degrees of pressure, areas of concentration, and body positions, but all strive to provide relaxation and improved conditioning of body tissues and fluids.
- While informal massage can provide both relaxation and a social outlet, genuine health benefits can be obtained by employing a positive intent and some knowledge of the underlying anatomy.

RESOURCES

▓ American Massage Therapy Association

www.amtamassage.org

▓ International Association of Infant Massage

www.iaim-us.com

▓ National Certification Board for Therapeutic Massage and Bodywork

www.ncbtmb.com

▓ Rolf Institute

www.rolf.org

In This Chapter

- The varieties of pressure-point therapy and their histories
- The systems and practice of pressure point therapies
- Putting pressure-point therapies to work for you

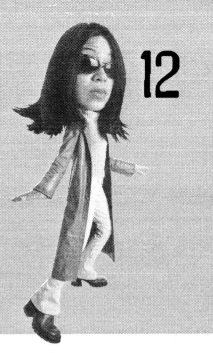

12

Pressure-Point Therapies

Acupuncture, acupressure, *Jin Shin Jyutsu*, *Jin Shin Do*, and reflexology are different forms of the same practice: stimulating points on the body to balance the body's life energy. Jin Shin Jyutsu, Jin Shin Do, and reflexology are forms of acupressure and in this chapter the term acupressure includes all the forms. Acupuncture and acupressure are based on the theory that applying pressure or stimulation to specific points on the body, known as acupuncture points, can relieve pain, cure certain illnesses, and promote wellness. Acupuncture uses needles while acupressure uses finger pressure. Although the older of the two techniques, acupressure is not as powerful and could be considered the over-the-counter version of acupuncture. Acupressure is easy to learn and convenient for self-care whereas acupuncture requires training to use the needles. Frequently, these practices are part of a holistic approach to wellness and are combined with diet, herbs, mind-body techniques, and spiritual therapies.

What Are Pressure Point Therapies?

Acupuncture and acupressure started in China several thousand years ago. The practice spread to Korea around 300 CE and to Japan in the seventeenth century. In the late nineteenth century a Canadian physician, Sir William Osler, became interested in acupressure techniques, but they remained largely unknown in North America until the 1970s. Accompanying President Richard Nixon on his trip to China in 1972, James Reston, a reporter for the *New York Times*, wrote about his experience with acupuncture for relief of pain following abdominal surgery in China. This article began the upsurge of interest in these therapies in the United States. Consumers in the United States have increasingly turned to acupuncture and acupressure to maintain their health and treat various disorders. They spend $500 million a year on acupuncture for complaints ranging from low-back pain to migraines to gallstones. Used with great success on humans for thousands of years, acupuncture and acupressure are now available for cats, dogs, and horses through veterinarians trained in Traditional Chinese Medicine.

Jin Shin Jyutsu (pronounced jin-shin JIT-soo) and *Jin Shin Do* are Japanese phrases meaning The Way of the Compassionate Spirit. They are ancient practices that fell into relative obscurity until they were dramatically revived in the early 1900s by Master Jiro Murai in Japan. Dying from a terminal illness, he turned in desperation to Jin Shin Jyutsu and meditation. Within a week he was completely well. He spent the remaining 50 years of his life researching and sharing his knowledge of this healing art, which he referred to as the art of happiness, the art of longevity, and the art of benevolence. After World War II, a Japanese American, Mary Burmeister, studied with Master Murai for many years and eventually returned to the United States with the "gift" of Jin Shin Jyutsu and Jin Shin Do. Today, thousands of students throughout the United States and around the world study and practice Jin Shin Jyutsu and Jin Shin Do.

Reflexology, an associated ancient practice, limits the use of acupressure points, or reflexes, to the feet, hands, and ears. William Fitzgerald, an American physician, introduced reflexology to the West in 1913. He noted that postoperative pain was less when pressure was applied to people's feet and hands just before surgery. In spite of Fitzgerald's work, it was the efforts of Eunice Ingham, a physical therapist, who expanded and refined Fitzgerald's observations and found that reflexology not only reduced pain but provided other health benefits as well. Ingham mapped the specific reflex zones on the feet, hands, and ears that reflexologists use today. This work gave her the distinction of being the founder of modern reflexology in the West.

The United States has more than 40 schools and colleges of acupuncture, 20 of which have either been approved or are currently being reviewed for approval by the National Accreditation Commission for Schools and Colleges of Acupuncture and Oriental Medicine. Thirty-two states regulate the practice of acupuncture, and of the 6,500 acupuncturists practicing in the United States, about 3,300 have taken the examination administered by the National Commission for the Certification of Acupuncturists (NCCA). To take the exam, candidates must have completed three years of full-time training and apprenticed with a certified acupuncturist for three years. Immigrant acupuncturists trained abroad must have practiced acupuncture for four years in lieu of apprenticeship.

An estimated 5,000 American doctors now include acupuncture in their practices. Most are family physicians, anesthesiologists, orthopedists, and pain specialists. Few physicians are NCCA-certified, but most are certified by the American Academy of Medical Acupuncture instead. Even though acupuncture is used in China to treat many conditions, in the United States conventional physicians have taken the technique out of context, using it most often to relieve acute and chronic pain. Nationally, an estimated 12,000 nonmedical doctors practice acupuncture, including nurses, naturopathic physicians, and chiropractors.

Professionals using acupressure are usually physical therapists or massage therapists with special training in this field. Some nurses are trained in acupressure and use it to help clients sleep and to reduce levels of anxiety. Midwives may use acupressure techniques to promote relaxation during labor and reduce breast engorgement after delivery. No specific license or certification is needed to practice any of the forms of acupressure.

How Do Pressure Point Therapies Work?

Like most alternative medicine, pressure point therapy regards health as a state of harmony, or balance, of the opposing forces of nature, both internal and environmental. The body requires balanced yin and yang energy to function properly and utilize its natural ability to resist disease. It is believed that everything you need to maintain and restore health already exists in nature and that pressure point therapies free up energy and restore balance, thus enabling individuals to maintain or regain their health.

Symptoms are caused by an imbalance of yin and yang in some part of the body, leading to excesses or deficiencies of life energy throughout the body. When the flow of energy becomes blocked or congested, people experience discomfort or pain on a physical level, may feel frustrated or irritable on an emotional level, and may experience a sense of vulnerability or lack of purpose in life on a spiritual level. When the flow of energy is interrupted, the area cannot nourish or cleanse. If not corrected, these blocks and imbalances in energy channels can result in disease and eventually illness.

The goal of care is to recognize and manage the disruption before illness or disease occurs. Qi can be thrown out of balance in a number of ways, including genetic vulnerability, accident or trauma, diet, lifestyle, emotional upset, spiritual distress, climate, or noxious agents. Pressure point practitioners bring balance to the body's energies, promoting optimal health and well-being and facilitating your own healing capacity.

Meridians

Acupuncture, acupressure, Jin Shin Jyutsu, Jin Shin Do, and reflexology are treatments rooted in the traditional Eastern philosophy that qi, or life energy, flows through the body along pathways known as meridians. Like major power lines, the meridians connect all parts of the body. As vital energy flows through the meridians, it forms tiny whirlpools close to the skin's surface at places called *hsueh*, which means cave or hollow. In Traditional Chinese Medicine, these are acupuncture points; in India, *marma* points. These pressure points function somewhat like gates to moderate the flow of qi. Acupuncture needles inserted into these points or pressure on these points releases blocked energy and improves the circulation of qi in the body.

The body has 14 major meridians and 360 to 365 classic points through which qi can be accessed. Most practitioners, however, focus on 150 points. The points themselves are metaphors for a person's journey through life with names such as "Spirit Gate," "Great Esteem," "Joining the Valleys," and "Inner Frontier Gate." Each meridian is also associated with an internal organ after which it is named: stomach, spleen, heart, small intestine, bladder, kidney, circulation–sex, gall bladder, liver, lung, and large intestine. The triple-warmer meridian is associated with the thyroid and adrenal glands, the governing meridian with the spine, and the central meridian with the brain. Chapter 3, "Traditional Chinese Medicine," presents more detailed information regarding energy and meridians.

Microsystems

At many points in the body the meridians converge. These points are reflexes to distant parts of the body and are called microsystems. *Microsystems* are areas of the body that are small, local representations of the whole body and are located on the feet, hands, and ears. In other words, each individual part of the body has an associated reflex on the ear, the hand, and the foot. The reflexes are symmetrical in that organs on the right side of the body are in the right foot, and the left organs on the left foot. The reflexes also correspond in descending order: The brain reflexes are in the tips of the toes, the eyes and ears under the toes, the shoulders and lungs on the ball of the foot, the stomach and pancreas on the instep, the intestines and colon towards the heel, and the hips on the heel. See Figures 12.1–12.3 for reflexology maps.

FIGURE 12.1

Diamonds on the soles of your feet: foot reflexology points.

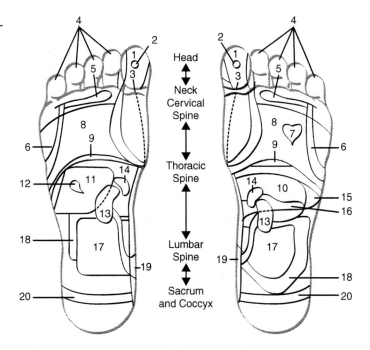

FIGURE 12.2

Your whole self in your hand: hand reflexology points.

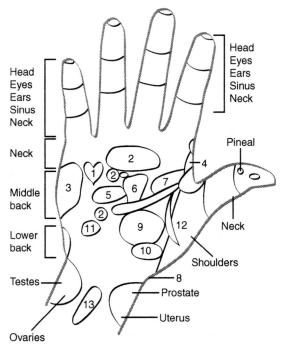

FIGURE 12.3

Now hear this: ear reflexology points.

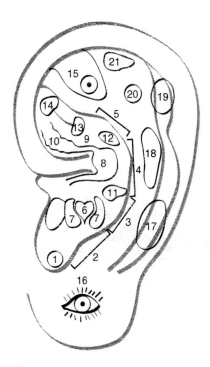

Mind-Body Connections

In the pressure point tradition, the mind, body, spirit, and emotions are never separated. Thus, the heart is not just a blood pump; the heart also influences your capacity for joy, sense of purpose in life, and connectedness with others. The kidneys filtrate fluids but they also manage your capacity for fear, will and motivation, and faith in life. The lungs breathe in air and breathe out waste products, but they also regulate your capacity to grieve, as well as acknowledgment of self and others. The liver cleanses the body, and it influences one's feeling of anger as well as that of vision and creativity. The stomach has a part in digestion of food and influences your ability to be thoughtful, kind, and nurturing as well. These are just a few of the mind-body connections that pressure point practitioners recognize.

What Happens During a Pressure-Point Session

The initial consultation involves a holistic assessment, because no part of the self is considered a neutral bystander when the body is in a state of imbalance. A detailed medical history is an important part of the diagnostic process. Special attention is paid to the connection between body, mind, emotions, and spirit.

If pressure point therapies are done within the context of Traditional Chinese Medicine, palpation is the major diagnostic method. Reading the pulses provides a remarkable amount of information about the person's condition. Imbalances in the body can be detected through palpating microsystems on the feet, hands, and ears. If something feels different in the microsystems, the corresponding organ is examined in more detail. Chapter 3 discusses the diagnostic process of Traditional Chinese Medicine in greater detail.

Pressure point therapies consider symptoms to be an expression of the condition of the person as a whole. Thus, sessions focus not only on relieving pain and discomfort, but also on responding to disruptions before they develop into illnesses.

Acupuncture

To restore the flow of energy, acupuncturists insert sterile, hair-thin needles at points along the meridians. The needles are rotated, twirled, or accompanied by a weak electrical current, and are often left in several minutes or longer. Acupuncturists also may apply heat or use finger pressure to alter the flow of qi. Clients feel little, if any, pain. Some people experience sensations of warmth, tingling, heaviness, or a dull ache.

Evidence now indicates that, in addition to restoring the flow of energy within the meridians, acupuncture reduces pain by triggering the release of endorphins. Acupuncture also stimulates the nervous system to release ACTH, a chemical that aids in fighting inflammation; it also releases prostaglandins, which help wounds heal more quickly, and other substances that may promote nerve regeneration. Unlike drugs and surgery, acupuncture has virtually no side effects.

Jin Shin Jyutsu/Jin Shin Do

Jin Shin Jyutsu/Jin Shin Do can be practiced by a trained practitioner or by you. The fingertips are placed over clothing on designated pressure points, to harmonize and restore the energy flow. Rather than doing something to the body, Jin Shin encourages the body to "let go," which is seen as the path to awakening your awareness of harmony within yourself and the universe.

A session generally lasts about an hour with the client lying on a table fully clothed. The practitioner's hands act as "jumper cables" to "kick start" the correct flow of energy. A spot on the shoulder may be held at the same time as a spot on the knee. The practitioner uses special sequences of hand positions to stimulate the circulation of energy. The touch is gentle, steady, and never involves force. It is generally pain-free; any tenderness in a particular area is caused by a blockage and tends to dissipate as the area is held. Some people may feel hot or cold or feel a sensation in another part of the body than where the practitioner is working. Most people experience a sense of deep relaxation with Jin Shin Jyutsu/Jin Shin Do.

Reflexology

Reflexologists manipulate the reflex zones most commonly on the feet but the hands or ears may also be manipulated. A session usually lasts about 45 minutes with the client sitting comfortably in a chair with the practitioner using thumb and fingers in small, creeping movements over the sole of the foot. This manipulation prompts the nervous system to speed up the body's response to an afflicted area by stimulating the flushing of toxins from the area.

Putting Pressure on Yourself: Therapies to Try at Home

Here are some simple techniques to help you work with your pressure points to relieve discomfort or pain. Once you think you have located one of the appropriate points, probe the area with a fingertip or pencil eraser in a tight circular motion in the general location. Points often feel tender, sore, or tingling. Press the point for one minute, then stop for a few seconds, and press again. Work the point for 5 to 20 minutes. If you are experiencing a headache, hiccups, or symptoms of carpal tunnel syndrome, experiment for yourself and find which points work best for you. Remember, only some of the points need to be worked to achieve relief.

caution

Pressure point therapy is not appropriate for every ailment!

People with acute or infectious illness, fever, or those needing surgery should seek conventional therapy. Foot injuries need to heal before the use of reflexology. Tell your practitioner if you have a pacemaker: They will avoid that area. Likewise, if you have gallstones or kidney stones, those areas should also be avoided. Finally, pressure point therapy is not recommended during pregnancy, as it may induce uterine contractions.

Headache

Point 1.   Hold your hand open, palm down, and find the point in the center of the fleshy webbing between the thumb and index finger.

Point 2.   Find the point on the top of the foot in the valley between the big toe and second toe.

Point 3.   Point number three is at the base of the back of the skull in the hollow above the two large vertical neck muscles.

Point 4.   This point is in the hollow above the inner eyes, where the bridge of the nose meets the ridge of the eyebrows.

Point 5.   Find the point between the eyebrows where the bridge of the nose meets the forehead.

Point 6.   This point is two finger-widths above the webbing of the fourth and fifth toes in the groove between the bones.

Hiccups

Point 1. Find the point in the indentation behind each earlobe.

Point 2. This point is located at the base of the throat in the center of the collarbone.

Point 3. Find this point on the center of the breastbone three thumb-widths up from the base of the bone.

Point 4. This point is located three finger-widths below the base of the breastbone in the pit of the abdomen. If you are healthy, do not press this point for more than two minutes. If you are not healthy, do not press this point at all.

Carpal Tunnel Syndrome

Point 1. Find the point in the middle of the inner side of the forearm, two and a half finger widths below the wrist crease.

Point 2. This point is located in the middle of the inside of the wrist crease.

Point 3. Find the point on the outside of the forearm, midway between the radius and ulna, two and a half finger widths below the wrist crease.

Foot Massage

When your feet ache, your whole body suffers. Here are instructions for a 10-to-15-minute foot massage to relax and soothe your feet and perhaps your entire body.

- Sit in a comfortable, quiet place where you will not be disturbed. You may want to have soothing music in the background.

- Pour a small amount of nongreasy lotion or massage oil into your hands and rub them together.

- Begin massaging one foot, stroking each toe in an up-and-down motion. Then massage the entire foot using kneading, wringing motions until the lotion is absorbed.

- Holding your foot firmly in one hand, press the thumb of the other hand (slightly bent) on the sole of the foot near the heel. Apply even pressure with the thumb and "walk it" forward, little by little. Press one spot, move forward, press again, move forward, and so on.

- When you get to the toes, go back to the heel and trace another line from heel to toe. Continue this process until the entire sole of the foot has been worked.

- Repeat the entire process with the other foot.

Accupressure of the Hand

To ease tension and restore energy, try this pressure point: hold your left palm in front of you, fingers together. The fleshy spot between your thumb and index finger is a key pressure point. Using your right thumb, massage this spot in a circular motion for a slow count of 15. Then switch hands, and repeat the process. You can also try several finger holds to improve your general level of well-being. Gently hold the appropriate finger on either hand while imaging the negative emotions melting away and the physical symptoms easing:

- Thumb. Corresponds to worrying, depression, anxiety. Physical symptoms may be stomachaches, headaches, skin problems, and nervousness.

- Index finger. Corresponds to fear, mental confusion, frustration. Physical symptoms are digestive problems and muscle problems such as backaches.

- Middle finger. Corresponds with anger, irritability, indecisiveness. Physical symptoms are eye or vision problems, fatigue, and circulation problems.

- Ring finger. Corresponds with sadness, fear of rejection, grief, negativity. Physical symptoms are digestive, breathing, or serious skin problems.

- Little finger. Corresponds with insecurity, effort, overdoing it, nervousness. Physical symptoms are sore throat and bone or nerve problems.

The Absolute Minimum

- All pressure-point therapies attempt to manipulate the body's energy field at points where the energy meridians are at or near the surface of the body

- Acupuncturists use hair-thin needles, acupressure therapists use touching and varying degrees of pressure on the body, and reflexologists concentrate their attention on the feet, hands, and ears.

- You can manipulate your own pressure points to find relief from some everyday aches and pains.

RESOURCES

- American Academy of Medical Acupuncture

  www.medicalacupuncture.org

- International Institute of Reflexology

  www.reflexology-usa.net

- Jin Shin Institute

  www.jinshininstitute.com

- National Certification Commission for Acupuncturists & Oriental Medicine

  www.nccaom.org

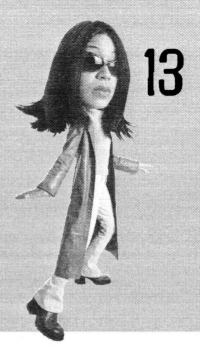

13

Energy-Balancing Therapies

A wide variety of alternative healing practices emerging in popularity are designed to balance the body's *biofield*, or energy field, and increase the flow of energy. Richard Gerber, M.D., author of *Vibrational Medicine*, defines biofield therapy or energy medicine as the emerging science of using various forms of energy for diagnosis and healing. Reviewing hundreds of research studies, Gerber hypothesizes that conscious and unconscious thoughts exist as energy that surrounds and permeates the body. While these studies are in their early stages, validation of the existence of the human energy field is beginning to emerge. More detailed discussion of the concept of body energy is found in Chapter 2, "How Does Alternative Medicine Work?"

What Are Energy-Balancing Therapies?

The three most prominent therapies using the hands to alter the body's energy field and impact the healing process are Therapeutic Touch (TT), Healing Touch (HT), and Reiki. All three approaches could be simply defined as the use of the hands on or near the body with the intention to help or to heal. Actually, the word touch is a misnomer in Therapeutic and Healing Touch, because the practitioner doesn't necessarily touch the recipient to achieve the desired effects during a healing session. Techniques are usually performed inches and sometimes feet from the recipient's body. These therapies are modern interpretations of several ancient healing practices, traditionally known as the "laying on of hands." TT, HT, and Reiki, however, must not be confused with faith healing, as the context in which they are practiced is not religious but scientific.

The goals of these hand-mediated therapies are to accelerate the person's own healing process and to facilitate healing at all levels of body, mind, emotions, and spirit. All three are forms of treatment and are not designed to diagnose physical conditions. Nor are they meant to replace conventional surgery, medicine, or drugs in treating organic disease.

Therapeutic touch is practiced by an estimated 40,000–50,000 American nurses. The brainchild of Dolores Krieger, R.N., Ph.D., of New York University, she launched the TT movement in 1970 after studying with Dora Kunz, a past president of the Theosophical Society of America and a natural healer. TT refers to the Krieger-Kunz Method of Therapeutic Touch, and was originally developed as an energy field interaction between nurse and client. Dr. Krieger, along with Janet Quinn, R.N., Ph.D., from the University of Colorado School of Nursing, has devoted her career to the research, study, and teaching of TT. TT has been taught in more than 80 universities and colleges in the United States and in more than 70 other countries–primarily in schools of nursing.

Healing touch refers to approaches taught in the American Holistic Nurses Association's (AHNA) Certificate Program in Healing Touch for Health Care Professionals. Healing-touch therapy was developed by Janet Mentgen, R.N., B.S.N., a Colorado nurse who has been practicing energy-based care since 1980. When Mentgen was introduced to TT, she added it to her extensive healing repertoire and created the Healing Touch approach. In 1990, her five-course sequence in HT became the first certified program offered by the AHNA.

Reiki is a Tibetan/Japanese technique for stress reduction, relaxation, and promotion of healing. The word Reiki is made of two Japanese words: rei, which means "God's Wisdom or the Higher Power," and ki, which is "life force energy." Thus Reiki means "spiritually guided life force energy." Reiki is an ancient Buddhist practice rediscovered by a Japanese physician, Dr. Usui, using ancient Tibetan texts. He first used

Reiki on himself and his family and then began to share his knowledge with the larger public. He opened a clinic in Tokyo in 1922 and his fame for healing spread quickly all over Japan. Reiki was introduced in the United States by Hawayo Takata, a Japanese-American woman, who studied with Dr. Usui.

The Education of Therapeutic Hands

Therapeutic Touch does not require extensive formal training. It can be learned by most anyone who is motivated by compassion and committed to helping others. Family members can be taught how to use it effectively with their loved ones. In fact, one of the leading researchers and teachers of this method, Janet Quinn, Ph.D., R.N., has created a videotape home-study course for family caregivers. (See the Resource section.)

Nurses who seek certification as Healing Touch practitioners from the AHNA are expected to do extensive reading, including books about techniques, healing traditions, self-healing, and possible theoretical explanations. The preparation may take two to three years of study. Most programs strongly emphasize "healer, heal thyself," and practitioners are encouraged to process their own issues.

Reiki is usually learned from a Reiki Master. There are two degrees in Reiki healing, as well as a Master degree that prepares one to teach others. Most people can complete the first degree in a weekend course. The content includes historical information, the concept of energy healing, how to transfer energy from oneself to another person, and the hand positions used in healing. The second degree, also done over a weekend, includes learning how to do distant healing and further enhancement of your physical, mental, emotional, and spiritual healing abilities. The Master degree takes years of additional study and a training mentorship with a Master Reiki practitioner.

How do Energy-Balancing Therapies Work?

By any name—*chi*, *ki*, *prana*, subtle energy—a life force energy is universally recognized in biofield therapies as the core of life and the driving force in healing. The belief is that all living beings are complex networks of interwoven vibratory fields surrounded by an energy field, and that energy centers within that biofield control the energy flow into and out of the body. It is at this level of the subtle energy system that both health and illness originate. Energy field theory is based on quantum physics theory, which posits that matter is energy and that all things generate vibratory fields interconnected by mathematical laws.

Although no adequate Western scientific evidence currently supports the existence of this human energy field, many of the most sophisticated instruments widely used in conventional medicine for diagnosis and treatment are energy-medicine devices. The electrocardiogram, electroencephalogram, electromyogram, ultrasound, and magnetic resonance imaging devices all measure the electromagnetic frequencies emitted by various parts of the body. Energy medicine is now used to heal bone fractures, relieve pain, reduce inflammation, and improve circulation. Chapter 23, "Bioelectromagnetics," covers this healing in greater detail. As scientists learn to recognize the subtler expressions of energy, old and new energy therapies will continue to complement the practice of conventional medicine.

People can detect a far greater spectrum of energies than can scientific measuring devices. Elmer Green of the Menninger Foundation believes that people's ability to sense and work with subtle energies is based in a communication system in the body that links the endocrine glands, nervous system, and the biofield. William Collinge, author of *Subtle Energy*, believes that many phenomena that are dismissed as coincidences—instances of extrasensory perception, *déjà vu*, and precognition—are part of a subtle perceptual system outside our five senses. He believes that everyone has the ability to sense energies that are not detectable with our current technology, but that many Western individuals reject their intuitive experiences because of a belief that anything that cannot be measured does not exist.

It is this energy field that skilled biofield practitioners can literally feel and modulate. The working hypotheses of TT are as follows:

- Human beings are energy fields.
- These energy fields are receptive to intentional repatterning.
- Trained practitioners may assist in the intentional repatterning of a recipient's energy field.

Researchers and proponents of TT believe an intention or strong wish to help the receiver is necessary as well as a conscious use of self as a link between the universal life energy and the other person. Prior to the actual intervention, practitioners focus completely on the well-being of the recipient in an act of unconditional love and compassion. Compassion, basic to all healing intervention, involves two things: intention and action. TT practitioners always set in mind their intention before entering and intervening in others' energy fields.

In the early days, most biofield therapists thought they acted solely as a conduit or a channel for environmental energy. Because people are open systems, the transfer of energy is a natural, continuous event. Therefore, it is conceivable that one person could transfer energy to another through conscious intent. That view has since been modified to include repatterning the recipients' energy systems by providing an example of a healthier pattern. When two people are in close proximity to one another, their energy fields overlap. As they intermingle, each energy field influences the other. Through close proximity or actual touch, two people create a larger, joint energy field by connecting their individual energy fields. In intentional healing situations, practitioners regulate their own internal energy frequencies, allowing recipients to draw upon the healers' resources and energy patterns. In an intentional healing situation, with or without physical contact, a state of coherence and synchrony between the brain waves of the healer and the recipient develops and they literally become unified in one energetic field.

Smoothing the Way for Healing

Within individuals, energy flows like a river. If it encounters no obstructions, it is smooth, gliding, and barely perceptible. People whose energy flows smoothly usually report good health and a feeling of peace with themselves and with others. Health, then, is defined as an abundance of *qi* and a balance or harmony of body, mind, and spirit. In addition, healthy people experience an equilibrium between their own energy systems and those of the environment. If obstructions or imbalance in energy occur, such as trauma, pain, rage, sadness, or any physical, mental, emotional, or spiritual problem, the balanced stream of energy is disrupted and illness or disease may result.

The locus of healing is within each person and cannot be "given" to a client by a biofield therapist. People must, and do, heal themselves. Healing environments are created when therapists enter into caring moments with clients. This moment provides a spirit-to-spirit connection in which the healer helps their clients to heal themselves. As recipients become engaged in the healing process, they often find new ways of coping with their illness.

TT, HT, and Reiki are used only as forms of treatment, not to diagnose physical conditions. They work in conjunction with other medical or therapeutic techniques to promote healing and relieve side effects of conventional therapies. Indications include irritability and anxiety; lethargy, fatigue, and depression; premenstrual syndrome; nausea and vomiting; chemotherapy and radiation sickness; wound and bone healing; and acute musculoskeletal problems such as sprains and muscle spasms. These healing practices are often effective in many types of pain. The only possible side effects of biofield therapies are temporary light-headedness and/or a temporary sensation of heat.

Practitioners believe that when they work with energy fields, they are dealing with that person as a whole and healing may occur at many levels. Recipients may experience emotional and spiritual growth as well as physical improvement, while in some cases the therapy may seem not to work at all. Even when these methods do not help people to resolve a particular problem, the session is soothing and relaxing.

EXPERIENCE YOUR ENERGY FIELD

- Vigorously rub your hands together for 20–30 seconds.
- Hold your palms together, parallel but not touching.
- Slowly separate them a couple of inches.
- Slowly bring them close together again.
- Repeat this process several more times, each time separating your palms by an additional two inches, until they are eight inches apart.
- You should be able to detect your energy field as you bring your palms together; you may feel a sense of bounciness, sponginess, or elasticity; some people describe it as the feeling of two magnets repelling each other.

The Experience of Energy-Balancing Healing

A third party witnessing a session between a patient and an energy-balancing healer might believe that nothing was really happening. The other two parties would surely beg to differ. The following descriptions of TT, HT, and Reiki sessions will help you better understand what's really happening during such a healing session.

Therapeutic Touch

Sessions of TT last up to 30 minutes and can be done with the patient sitting or lying down, fully clothed. Practitioners often combine both physical and nonphysical contact during the course of treatment. It is not necessary, however, to touch the physical body, which makes this technique especially helpful in situations where the person may not be able to tolerate contact, such as with burn victims or in the case of acute rheumatoid arthritis. Patients do not have to believe in the efficacy of TT to receive benefit. The one absolutely essential ingredient in TT, however, is the goodwill and compassion of the practitioner.

The first step in the TT process is centering, which is performed by the practitioner before beginning the actual treatment. *Centering* is a general term for any method that people use to quiet themselves physically, mentally, and emotionally. Centering can be achieved by many methods, such as deep breathing, visualization, and focusing, which allow the practitioner to relax and focus on the intent of the healing session. Being centered allows healers to operate intuitively, with awareness, and to channel energy throughout their bodies. The sidebar, "Centering Yourself," describes one centering method.

CENTERING YOURSELF

- Sit or stand comfortably and close your eyes or focus on one spot on the floor.
- Breathe in and out, slowly and deeply, concentrating on how the breath feels as it goes in and out.
- Breathe in relaxation and peace while breathing out stress and tension.
- Imagine a fairly large tree; really sense the tree as it sounds, as it smells, and according to the season.
- Get close to the tree and put your hands on the tree; lean up against the tree and put your full weight on the tree.
- Look up through the branches and feel the sun shining down; feel the sun traveling down through the tree and coming in through your head, down through your body, and out your legs.
- Focus once again on your breathing and know that you can come back to this place at any time.
- With practice and experience, you will be able to center yourself within one or two deep breaths.

Once centered, the practitioner uses their hands to assess the recipient's energy field. The hands are positioned two to six inches from the body and, beginning at the head, are smoothed over the face, side and back of the head, and shoulders, as if smoothing out a piece of fabric. The assessment continues down the body and over both legs. Some are able to feel the energy field when they first learn TT, while for others it takes months of practice to experience the sensations. Different people describe different sensations commonly characterized as heat, cold, tingling, buzzing, emptiness, or pressure. The energy field is assessed for bilateral similarities or differences in the flow of energy. A healthy energy field is symmetrical with a smooth, flowing texture.

The next step in TT is clearing and balancing the energy field. Again, the hands are moved in a flowing motion two to six inches from the body. Blocked areas of energy are moved by using slow brushing motions from the top down and away from the body. This motion is repeated until the practitioner no longer feels the blockage and the energy is moving freely and easily. This step typically lasts for 5 to 15 minutes.

Direction of energy is the next step in TT. Depending on the particular problem, the practitioners will consciously focus their attention and intention on slowing the energy flow, stimulating the energy flow, or reestablishing the rhythm of the energy flow in problem areas. This redirection is done by placing one hand on the recipient's middle back at the level of the kidneys while holding the other hand two to three inches in front of the corresponding area on the abdomen. Practitioners visualize universal energy entering their bodies through their feet or their crown chakras. This healing energy then moves through their body, pouring out through the hand that is on the recipient's back, and flowing through the recipient's body to the hand on the front of the abdomen. This process lasts as long as it is comfortable or effective, typically for 5 to 15 minutes. The ending phase of TT is similar to the beginning phase as the hands are swept over the body from head to toe, smoothing out the energy field. The treatment session often ends in helping clients "ground" or become aware of their current physical experience. Often it is accomplished by gently holding the tops of both feet for a minute or two.

Healing Touch

The process of an HT session is usually similar to TT, though more emphasis is placed on the practitioner's intuition and its role in working out the problems in the client's energy field. Treatment time will therefore be more variable than in TT. Practitioners generally use their hands to assess the recipient's energetic state. The goal is to smooth the flow of energy, to mobilize it if stuck, and to leave the client with an energy flow that feels smooth, powerful, and unobstructed. HT techniques are developed intuitively and derived from various approaches such as TT, Native American medicine, and other energy healing modalities. HT treatments might last as little as five minutes or as long as necessary, depending on the problem, the technique chosen, the practitioner's skill, and the recipient's response.

Reiki

A Reiki session typically lasts one hour and consists of practitioners channeling universal life-force energy to the clients. The goal is to restore balance in the client's energy field. During sessions, practitioners lay their hands on or above a specific problem area while transferring universal life energy to the recipient. A series of 15 hand positions are designed to cover all body systems. Each hand position is held for five minutes or until the flow of energy is reestablished.

How Can I Get Started with Energy-Balancing Therapy?

In the current health care environment, people with acute and chronic disorders are rapidly discharged back to the community. Family and friends are often overwhelmed by caregiver responsibilities. Often they feel helpless in the face of their loved one's obvious suffering or pain. Learning TT can be a powerful tool to help counteract the sense of helplessness that can be experienced. As caregivers discover that TT can minimize the experience of pain and increase the sense of relaxation, they often feel they have something "worthwhile" to offer. In addition, the use of TT can be helpful to the caregiver, who is most likely exhausted from trying to carry on the normal daily routine, as well as care for the sick or injured person. Because the first step of TT is centering, the process demands that caregivers take a few minutes for themselves as they concentrate on their own well-being and sense of peace. As caregivers increase their self-awareness, they are quicker to recognize tension and stress in their bodies, which, hopefully, encourages them to develop stress management skills. Dr. Janet Quinn has also made a TT videotape for caregivers, which is straightforward and easy to learn.

TT, HT, and Reiki produce a sense of well-being and relaxation for both the practitioner and the recipient. For some healers, it is the first time they have been given permission to be quiet, take a breath, and center during working hours. For some patients, this is their first encounter with a healer who has done so. When the healer is in a peaceful state of mind, that gentleness and kindness permeates the environment. Patients react positively to the treatments, but also to the individual attention from healers as they build relationships, offer noninvasive nurturing touch, and reduce stress and anxiety.

THE ABSOLUTE MINIMUM

- Energy-balancing therapies attempt to bring calmness and order to the energy fields believed to be created by and around every person.
- The key ingredients of balancing therapy are a healing intent and an openness to perceiving forces and conditions not readily apparent to the five senses.
- The practice of energy-balancing therapies is by no means limited to health-care professionals, and is a great way for those close to people with illnesses to play a role in the healing process.

RESOURCES

- Colorado Center for Healing Touch

    www.healingtouch.net

- Therapeutic Touch

    www.therapeutic-touch.org

- International Center for Reiki Training

    www.reiki.org

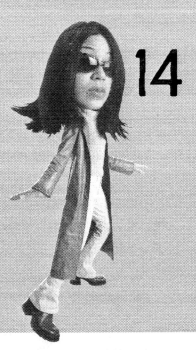

14

COMBINED MANUAL THERAPIES

The two methods described in this chapter, Applied Kinesiology and Polarity Therapy, are a combination of physical and energy-balancing interventions. Applied Kinesiology is both a diagnostic method and treatment that uses energy, lymphatic, neurovascular, and muscle systems. Polarity Therapy, a nondiagnostic healing system, is based on the theories of Traditional Chinese Medicine and Ayurvedic medicine and combines bodywork, diet, exercise, and counseling in the treatment of clients.

What Are Combined Therapies?

Applied Kinesiology was developed in the 1960s by George Goodheart and Alan G. Beardell, American chiropractic physicians. In the 1970s, John Thie, also a chiropractor, took their work, simplified it for the general public, and called this modified approach "Touch for Health." Polarity Therapy is a system of health care developed in the 1920s by an Austrian-American holistic physician, Randolph Stone, who was a chiropractor, osteopath, and naturopath. He studied and tested health theories from around the world, combining ancient and modern techniques. His first work was published in 1947, and by 1954 he had completed the seven books that contain his findings.

Health care professionals may go on to study Applied Kinesiology only after completion of their basic professional education. Applied Kinesiology is practiced by chiropractors, nurses, osteopaths, naturopaths, dentists, or physicians. Interested professionals take the training in a post-graduate setting, usually in weekend classes. The basic course takes more than 100 hours of classroom study and numerous hours of practice in the clinical setting after which students can test for basic proficiency. Another 200 hours of classes and the writing of at least two research papers are required to reach the next step, where written and oral exams are given. Organized courses in Applied Kinesiology are taught in Europe, Canada, the United States, and Australia. There is no licensure per se, and providers of Applied Kinesiology practice on their professional license.

Polarity Therapy is practiced by a variety of health care professionals who have completed their basic education. To achieve the level of Associate Polarity Practitioner, the applicant must take 155 classroom and clinical hours of study. Those wishing to become Registered Polarity Practitioners must take an additional 460 hours of study for cumulative hours totaling 615. No licensure is available at the present time. Some states, however, are considering licensing polarity therapists under massage therapists, even though they are distinct therapeutic practices.

How Do Combined Therapies Work?

As in many alternative practices, the concept of energy is at the heart of Applied Kinesiology and Polarity Therapy. The belief is in a life force of subtle energy that surrounds and permeates all living things, often referred to as a biofield. It is unclear at this time whether the biofield is electromagnetic or a field currently unknown to physics. The present hypotheses are that the biofield is a form of bioelectricity, biomagnetism, or bioelectromagnetism. The exact nature is not yet established and some researchers deny the reality of a biofield.

REDIRECTING THE FLOW OF ENERGY

Sit facing a partner and, placing both hands in the air, move your hands close to your partner's hands without touching. Experiment with distance and where you can feel the energy pulsating between your hands. Imagine that your partner's energy is coming in your left hand from your partner's right hand and your energy is flowing out your right hand into your partner's left hand. Imagine the circular circuit between the two of you as the energy flows up the left arm, across the heart, and down the right arm. Imagine how connected you feel at this given moment.

Meridians

Applied Kinesiology works closely with the meridian system and pressure points. Meridians are a network of energy circuits that run vertically through the body. Each meridian passes close to the skin's surface at places called pressure points. Since each meridian is associated with an internal organ, the points offer surface access to the internal organ system. Each of the 14 meridians has related specific neurovascular points and neurolymphatic points.

Neurovascular Points

Neurovascular points are located mainly on the head. A few seconds after placing one's fingers on these points, a slight pulse can be felt at a steady rate of 70–74 beats per minute. This pulse is not related to the heartbeat, but is believed to be the primitive pulsation of the microscopic capillary bed in the skin.

Neurolymphatic Points

The lymphatic system in the body flows only in one direction and acts as a drainage system of the body. It produces antibodies, makes white blood cells, and transports fats, proteins, and other substances to the blood system. The energy for the lymphatic system is regulated by neurolymphatic reflexes, located mainly on the chest and back. These reflex points act like switches that get turned off when the system is overloaded. They are usually tender spots and those reflex points which are the sorest are in greatest need of massage.

Polarity

The term polarity refers to the universal pulsation of expansion/contraction or attraction/repulsion known as yin and yang energy in Traditional Chinese Medicine. These polarized forces together make up the whole of anything. For example, all tissues in your body can be understood in terms of charged energy categorized as positive, negative, or neutral. These three energy types are in constant dynamic tension with each other, creating the basis for health or illness. Polarity between different body parts appears to be equivalent to polar differences in electromagnetic fields. Polarity therapists think of the right hand as the giving energy hand and the left as the receiving energy hand. It is believed that energy is affected and possibly distorted by life experiences and that these distortions may be corrected by a variety of healing methods.

What Is a Combined Therapy Session Like?

Well-being and health are determined by the nature of the flow of energy within and outside the body. When energy flows smoothly without significant blockage or fixation, the person experiences health in an ongoing and dynamic way. Disease and pain occur when energy is blocked, fixed, or unbalanced. When your physical body, thoughts, and emotions are out of alignment with the energy necessary to meet a life challenge, an energy imbalance results. Within the Applied Kinesiology framework, one of the signs of an imbalance is a weakening of the muscles and a change in the posture. If these minor problems are not corrected, the imbalances may develop into physical, mental, and emotional discomfort or pain. Pain and discomfort are seen as signals to people to learn, change, and realign their lives.

Diagnosis and Treatment

An Applied Kinesiology exam depends on knowledge of functional neurology, anatomy, physiology, biomechanics, and biochemistry. It is combined with standard procedures, laboratory findings, and x-rays and history taking. Generally, problems can be related to chemical imbalance, structural imbalance, mental stress, or any combination of these states. General examination procedures are used to assess the health of the client and are followed by specific examination procedures such as testing reflexes or assessing clients' balance.

Every muscle in the body is related to a specific organ or gland through the sharing of lymphatic vessels or meridians. Because organs and glands have few pain and sensory fibers, people are largely unaware of energetic imbalances in these parts. Unbalanced organs or glands, however, refer pain externally to the corresponding surface meridians and muscles indicating the cause of the problem. For example, the deltoid muscle in the shoulder shares a relationship with the lungs. If a person has abnormal lung function, such as bronchitis, pneumonia, congestion, or the flu, the problem may exhibit as a weakness in one or both deltoid muscles. When the lung problem is cleared up, the deltoid muscle returns to a normal state.

Manual testing of the 576 muscles of the body is done to augment the other examination procedures. Muscle weaknesses are often so subtle that physical therapists would consider the muscle strength to be within normal limits. No more than 15 percent difference should be discernable between the right and left sides. The testing positions are intended to isolate the muscle from the group with which it normally works, making it less strong than if it were used in the usual way. Small children, the elderly, and the frail will not be as strong as a healthy adult. It is more difficult to test a person who has great strength, such as an athlete, because the weakness is too difficult to be distinguished by the tester.

A number of causes result in weak muscles, including immobility, lack of exercise, poor posture, gland/organ dysfunction, dysfunction of the nerve supply, impairment of lymphatic drainage, decreased blood supply, blockage of meridians, and chemical imbalance. Testing of individual muscles is combined with knowledge of the basic mechanics and physiological functioning of the body to provide practitioners with information necessary to formulate a diagnosis.

Applied Kinesiology and Polarity Therapy practitioners believe that the body, mind, emotions, and spirit are interdependent. It is believed that people are responsible for their own health and that they can take simple steps to improve and maintain their level of wellness. The practitioner's role is to facilitate and support the client's self-healing capabilities.

Applied Kinesiology

Applied Kinesiology uses various methods to strengthen those muscles and related organs that were found to be weak during the diagnostic phase. Improvement in the flow of energy can be measured by increased muscle strength, which is assumed to lead to an increase in energy to the corresponding organs.

Neurovascular holding points are located mainly on the head. The practitioner makes simple contact with the pads of the fingers for anywhere from 20 seconds to 10 minutes, depending on the severity of the problem. This method appears to improve the blood circulation to both the muscle and the related organ, and the weak muscle will have increased strength when retested.

Neurolymphatic points are located mainly on the chest and back. Practitioners work on the points that are related to a specific weakened muscle by a deep massage of the points for 20–30 seconds. This massage is believed to turn on the blocked reflexes, allowing the lymph flow to return to normal. The weak muscle will have improved in strength when retested. Figure 14.1 illustrates the neurolymphatic points for the lungs.

Meridians are traced in the designated direction using both sides of the body. Practitioners use the flat of their hands to give better coverage. It can be done over clothing without actually touching the client. Tracing the meridian adds the practitioner's flow of energy to the recipient's energy in a blocked meridian and may restore the normal flow of energy. Figure 14.1 also illustrates the lung meridian.

FIGURE 14.1

Lung meridian and neurolymphatic holding points.

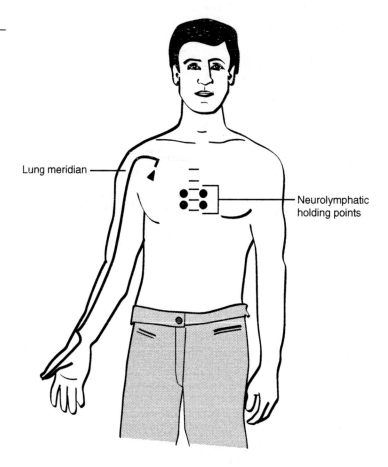

Lung meridian

Neurolymphatic holding points

Acupressure points are held on the same side of the body as the muscle that is weak. The first arm and leg points are held at the same time, one with each hand. Light pressure is maintained for about 30 seconds or until a pulse is felt in the leg. The hands are then moved to the second acupressure points and held, again waiting for the pulse in the leg. Figure 14.2 illustrates the pressure points for the lungs.

FIGURE 14.2

Acupressure points for the lungs.

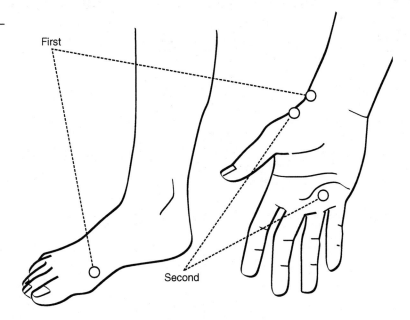

First

Second

Polarity Therapy

In a typical Polarity Therapy session, the practitioner assesses energy flow using palpation, observation, and interview with the recipient clothed for the entire session. Sessions usually take 60–90 minutes and involve both touch and verbal interaction. Touch contact may be light, medium, or firm and is used to stimulate and balance the body's biofield. During the session, the practitioner supports the client in increasing self-awareness of subtle energy sensations, which may be experienced as tingling, warmth, or wavelike movement. Clients are also helped to process feelings and develop specific strategies for reducing stress and increasing wellness. Clients are encouraged to take responsibility for their lives and create positive thinking that is the cornerstone of good health.

Both Applied Kinesiology and Polarity Therapy believe that nutrition plays a major role in health and well-being. Kinesiology assesses people's nutritional status, including food intolerances, vitamin and mineral deficiencies, and other chemical sensitivities. Polarity nutrition views food as energy and develops an ongoing, changing nutritional awareness rather than a rigid set of rules. Many practitioners support the value of a vegetarian diet with no meat, fish, fowl, or eggs. They also advocate periodic use of a "cleansing diet," consisting of fresh and cooked vegetables, as well as herbal cleansing practices and formulas.

Exercise is an important part of these therapies. Applied Kinesiology practitioners encourage clients to walk for exercise. Walking is one of the few exercises that benefits all parts of the body. All of the muscles are flowing when people walk with their arms swinging. Polarity yoga is a series of simple self-help energy techniques that create relaxation and balance. This body work includes gentle rocking and stretching postures combining breath and self-massage, both of which affect the flow of energy.

Applied Kinesiology can relieve pain, stress, and muscular disorders. It is used to detect allergies, nutritional deficiencies, back or neck pain, fatigue, headache, tension, and the common cold and is believed to have some benefit for those with learning disorders. Polarity Therapy induces profound relaxation, new insight into energy flow patterns, and relief from some physical problems.

EMOTIONAL FIRST AID

The next time you are upset try this procedure to decrease your stress.

- Hold your frontal eminences on your forehead either with the first two fingers of your hands—the right and left at the same time—or place the palm of your hand flat on your forehead.

- While applying light pressure, in your mind go over exactly what you are thinking and how you are feeling about the problem. Continue holding these points and going over what is bothering you for a few minutes or until you feel the emotions becoming less strong.

- Let go with your hands and look around you. Mentally review the issue again. If stressful feelings are still there or have changed to other stressful feelings (fear changed to anger, for example) go back and begin the process again.

The Absolute Minimum

- Applied Kinesiology and Polarity Therapy use a combination of physical and energy manipulation to restore the balance and flow of a patient's energy field.

- These therapies use concepts and techniques from many other types of alternative therapies, including energy meridians, acupressure, and the importance of nutrition and preventive health maintenance.

Resources

- American Polarity Therapy Association

  www.polaritytherapy.org

- Touch for Health Kinesiology Association

  www.tfh.org

PART V

Mind-Body Techniques

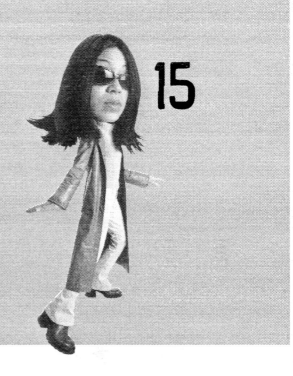

15

YOGA

Yoga has been practiced for thousands of years in India, where it is a way of life that includes ethical models for behavior and mental and physical exercises aimed at producing spiritual enlightenment. Although yoga developed from Hinduism, it is not a religion—but rather a journey of the body, mind, and spirit on a path toward unity. It is a method for life that can complement and enhance any system of religion, or it can be practiced completely apart from religion.

What Is Yoga?

The word *yoga* means to direct and concentrate one's attention, and comes from the Sanskrit word *yuj*, to yoke or to join. Yoga was first described by Patanjali, an Indian sage, who wrote the *Yoga Sutra* thousands of years ago. The Yoga Sutra recorded information that had been passed down orally for many years. This text has helped to define and shape the modern practice of yoga. Yoga first came to the United States in the 1890s, when Swami Vivekananda became a popular teacher and guide. In the 1960s, the Maharishi Mahesh Yoga, the creator of Transcendental Meditation, became a popular figure for America's "hippie generation," and the vogue has continued to grow since then.

The Western approach to yoga tends to be more fitness-oriented, while the Eastern approach to yoga is to prepare people for the experience of self-realization. Most Westerners begin yoga with the goal of managing their stress, learning to relax, and increasing their vitality and well-being. After learning yoga, many become more interested in the underlying principles of physical fitness and keeping the mind focused, calm, and clear. Yoga is meant to prepare the body and mind for a useful, dedicated life.

Much More Than Headstands

The various methods of yoga all have the same goal: to attain a state of pure bliss and oneness with the universe. *Raja* Yoga emphasizes control of the intellect to attain enlightenment, accomplished through meditation, concentration, and breath control. *Kriya* Yoga is the practice of quieting the mind through scriptural study, breath control, mantras, and meditation. *Karma* Yoga focuses on service to all beings as the path to enlightenment. *Bhakti* Yoga emphasizes devotion to the divine. *Inana* Yoga's goal is wisdom and the direct knowledge of the divine. *Tantra* Yoga involves the study of sacred writings and rituals. *Mantra* Yoga is the study of sacred sounds. *Kundalini* Yoga is the study of energy movement along the spine.

Although these many branches of yoga exist, this chapter focuses on *Hatha* Yoga as the form of yoga most frequently practiced by Westerners. In this particular type of yoga, the path to enlightenment is through control over the physical body as the key to control of the mind and freedom of the spirit. Physical exercises, breath control, and meditation tone and strengthen the whole person—body, mind, and spirit.

Eight Paths to Self-Realization

Classical yoga incorporates eight limbs or paths that provide structure for one's daily life. These physical and psychological practices are believed to contribute to a higher level of personal development. The outer aspect of yoga consists of right living (abstinence and personal discipline), right care of the body (body control), and enhancement of vital energy (breath control). Yoga also has an inner dimension that is the key purpose of yoga. Detachment, concentration, and meditation together form a single process toward the development of pure consciousness.

THE EIGHT LIMBS OF YOGA: GUIDELINES FOR LIVING

1. Abstinences (*yamas*)
   - Nonviolence (*ahimsa*)
   - Truthfulness (*satya*)
   - Nonstealing (*asteya*)
   - Chastity or nonlust (*brahmacharya*)
   - Nongreed (*aparigraha*)
2. Personal Disciplines (*niyamas*)
   - Purity (*shauca*)
   - Contentment (*santosha*)
   - Self-discipline (*tapas*)
   - Self-study (*svadhyaya*)
   - Centering on the divine (*ishvara-pranidhana*)
3. Body Control (*asanas*)
4. Breath Control (*pranayama*)
5. Detachment (*pratyahara*)
6. Concentration (*dharana*)
7. Meditation (*dhyana*)
8. Pure Consciousness (*samadhi*)

The Path of Abstinence

Abstinences are about what not to do in life. The first abstinence is about nonviolence. Nonviolence not only means not physically hurting others but also having nonviolent words and nonviolent thoughts. Truthfulness, the second abstinence, results in personal integrity and strength of character. Nonstealing, the third abstinence, includes not stealing other's material belongings as well as not taking credit for things one has not done, not stealing the center of attention, and so forth. The fourth abstinence, chastity or nonlust, means holding people in high esteem and loving and respecting others. The fifth abstinence is nongreed, which means living simply and viewing possessions as tools to use in life. Nongreed leads to the avoidance of jealousy and envy.

The Path of Personal Discipline

Personal disciplines are about what to do in life. Purity, the first discipline, is achieved through the practice of the five abstinences. The abstinences clear away negative ways of being, leading one straight to purity. Purity also relates to cleanliness and respect for all life. Contentment, the second discipline, means finding happiness with whom you are and with what you have. The third discipline, self-discipline, involves making a commitment and sticking to it. The fourth discipline, self-study, means self-examination through introspection. Centering on the divine, the fifth discipline, involves devotion. These disciplines work with any religion because individuals are encouraged to focus on how the divine is in them, part of them, and all around them.

The Path of Body Control

Body control, an important part of Hatha Yoga, is attained through a number of poses or *asanas*. These body positions are what most Westerners think of when they hear the word yoga. These poses help people learn to control their bodies, making them stronger, more flexible, better functioning, and more resistant to disease and other problems. Poses are also meant to facilitate meditation. The poses are frequently classified into the following groups: standing poses, inverted poses, twists, backward bending poses, forward bends, and poses for restoration. Another way of classifying poses is balance, strength, flexibility, and relaxation. The belief in nonviolence also applies to the poses, which means that physical exercise is never practiced to the point of pain, because pain is indicative of doing violence to the body.

The Path of Breath Control

Breath control teaches people to direct energy or *prana* for optimal physical and mental benefit. When air is inhaled, so is vital energy that flows into the body to nourish and enliven it. The purpose of balancing the breath is to make respiratory rhythm more regular, which in turn has a soothing effect on the entire nervous system. It also helps with meditation, because it focuses attention inward and reduces scattered thinking.

The Path of Detachment

The practice of detachment is the conscious withdrawal of the senses from everything that stimulates them. The goal of detachment is to gain mastery over external influences. This detachment can happen during breathing exercises, during meditation, or while doing the poses. The process of detachment can also be an effective technique for pain control.

The Path of Concentration

Teaching the mind to focus on one thing instead of many is the goal of concentration. Concentration is sustaining attention while at the same time quieting the mind and relaxing the breathing. Frequently people focus on one object such as a candle flame, the image of a circle, or a single sound. The purpose is to learn to push away the many thoughts that usually float around in one's mind. Concentration works directly on the body, allowing each yoga pose to accomplish the maximum possible benefit.

The Path of Meditation

Breath control, detachment, and concentration lead to the state of meditation. Meditation occurs when people become absorbed into the object on which they are concentrating. At this point, nothing else exists. It is through this process of meditation that you can clear your mind of clutter and thus think more quickly and see things more clearly in daily life. (This topic is explored more thoroughly in Chapter 16, "Meditation.")

The Golden Path of Pure Consciousness

The other seven limbs of yoga lead to pure consciousness, which produces a total merging with the object of meditation and, in such a way, becoming one with the universe. Generally speaking, it is "mind without thought." Many religions throughout history have pure consciousness as part of their tradition. Christianity refers to it as "pure love" and Judaism as the "divine nothingness" or "the naught." It is more than a mental or emotional experience. Physically, breathing slows drastically, the heart rate drops, and EEGs demonstrate unique patterns unlike any of the other three common states of consciousness—waking, sleeping, or dreaming. It is an ideal state, a state of pure bliss, and it is elusive for most people. A few rare and diligent yogis have been able to maintain this state for extended periods of time. Most others get occasional glimpses of it while meditating.

The Nature of Yogic Health

In yoga, health is related to the Five Sheaths of Existence. The first sheath is the physical body; the second is the vital body, life force, or prana; the third sheath is the mind, including thoughts and emotions; the fourth sheath is the higher intellect; and the fifth sheath is bliss, filled with positive energy and inner peace. It is believed that imbalances in any of these sheaths can result in illness. For example, intense anger, a disturbance in the third sheath, disrupts one's breathing pattern, which leads to an imbalance in prana or life force. The disrupted breathing allows the invasion of a virus leading to a disruption in the first sheath, manifesting as a cold. Living one's life in moderation is thought to keep all five sheaths in balance, which contributes to health and well-being.

Yogic thought places food or *ahara* on three levels. The first is the physical food that nourishes the body. The second is impressions or the sensations of sound, touch, sight, taste, and smell that nourish the mind. The third level is associations or the people who nourish the soul. Health and well-being are withdrawal from wrong food, wrong impressions, and wrong associations, while simultaneously opening up to the right food, right impressions, and right associations. Just as a healthy body resists toxins and pathogens, a healthy mind resists the negative influences around it.

The yogic perspective of health and illness is related to internal and external balance. Although it is recognized that viruses, bacteria, genetics, and accidents can cause illness, disorders can also be brought on by the following conditions:

- Insufficient prana, or life force
- Blocked prana
- Inappropriate diet
- Lack of cleanliness
- Unhappiness
- Pessimism and negativity

Healthy habits, maintenance of the body, peacefulness of mind, and calmness of spirit protect people from ill health. Yoga is a great preventive medicine. It helps the body cleanse itself of toxins by removing obstacles to the proper flow of the lymphatic system. Lymph is pumped through the body by movement—musculoskeletal movement, respiratory movement, circulatory movement, gastrointestinal movement, and so forth, all of which are part of yoga. Yoga also increases the flow of vital energy throughout the body by opening up and increasing the flexibility of body joints, considered to be minor chakras. Yoga poses and breathing techniques allow energy and lymph to flow freely through the entire body, resulting in a body that works better, feels better, and fights disease more effectively. Health, from a yogic perspective, can be described as the body easeful, the mind peaceful, and the life useful.

How Does Yoga Work?

In the West, most yogic practice is focused on hatha yoga, the search for enlightenment through control over the physical body. The regular practice of hatha yoga prepares the body and spirit for the exploration of all the paths of yoga. You can do as much or as little yoga as you wish. Some start with all three practices—poses, breath control, and meditation. Others start with the poses and may or may not develop interest in breathing and meditation.

As practiced in the United States, a typical yoga session lasts 20 minutes to an hour. Some sessions can spend 30 minutes doing poses and another 30 minutes doing breathing practices and meditation. Other sessions spend the majority of the time doing poses and end with a short meditation or relaxation procedure. Some people practice one to three times a week in a class, while others practice daily at home. Yoga should not be done within one to two hours after a heavy meal for the sake of abdominal comfort when doing the poses. Caffeine, and other stimulants, should be avoided because they may interfere with the goal of relaxation. Yoga should never be done under the influence of alcohol or recreational drugs, as they may decrease concentration, coordination, and strength, thus increasing the risk of physical injury. Yoga is best done in comfortable, loose clothing using a nonslippery surface like a rug, mat, or blanket. Since it is important that the process have your full attention, the room should be void of all extraneous noise, even soft background music.

Yoga is tailored to the individual and you can achieve great benefit at the beginner level as well as at the most advanced level. Participants must remember that yoga is not a competitive sport and thus a person's level does not matter. If people are stiff and out of shape, sick, or weak, sets of easy exercises can help loosen the joints and stimulate circulation. If practiced regularly, these simple exercises alone make a great difference in health and well-being.

Poses can be slow and careful or more vigorous. Beginning poses are used to relax tension in the muscles and joints and center the mind. Attention is paid to how the body feels and what it is doing. Every movement is made gently and slowly. Strain or force is to be avoided because yoga is a nonviolent approach that is performed comfortably. Strength training is isometric as the muscles are tensed in opposition to each other. After one assumes the pose, it is held for as long as possible comfortably, usually about six breaths. Each pose, in a well-structured workout, includes a pose and its opposite, such as a forward bend and a backward bend, so the body stays physically balanced. Breathing should be easy, fluid, and continuous and used to facilitate the poses.

Every yoga session should end with a few minutes of complete and total relaxation. This period is an important part of bringing the mind and body together to maximize the benefits. Some people end the session with chanting to reach a deeper state of relaxation.

Yoga offers a number of health benefits with virtually no risk of injury. The physical and psychological benefits include the following:

- Increases flexibility of muscles and joints
- Tones and strengthens muscles
- Improves endurance

- Increases circulation
- Lowers blood pressure
- Increases lymph circulation
- Improves digestion and elimination
- Promotes deeper breathing
- Increases brain endorphins, enkephalins, and serotonin
- Increases mental acuity
- Augments alpha and theta brain wave activity
- Promotes relaxation
- Manages stress

Yoga is not a cure-all for disease. It can help, however, to relieve symptoms, decrease pain, and improve the quality of life. It helps prevent disease by reinforcing lifestyle changes such as positive health habits and attitudes.

How Do I Begin a Yoga Practice?

The regular practice of yoga builds and tones muscles, increases flexibility, improves endurance, and promotes a state of relaxation. The physiologic responses are the opposite of the fight-or-flight stress response. Stretching and deep breathing bring on a profound sense of relaxation. Gentle stretching and range of motion joint exercises decrease muscle tension and joint stiffness. The mindful focus on awareness of self, breath, and energy minimizes anxiety associated with stress. Just getting your body down on the floor tends to clear the mind. Perhaps it is because being on the floor is so unusual to us that it changes our attitude toward and our awareness of our body. Yoga, combined with a low-fat diet and moderate aerobic exercise, can significantly reduce blockages in coronary arteries. Other studies have shown yoga to be effective in treating arthritis, diabetes, mood disorders, asthma, hypertension, menstrual cramps, back pain, and chronic fatigue.

Hatha yoga is designed by and for healthy, flexible people. Even when experiencing a serious illness, however, most people can work on breath control even if they do not feel up to doing the poses. The breathing exercises and relaxation response nourish the body, quiet the mind, and contribute to a more balanced state. Before beginning a yoga practice, you should check with your primary care practitioner if you have recently had surgery, have a debilitating physical handicap, or have cancer, diabetes, epilepsy, heart disease, high blood pressure, HIV, multiple sclerosis, or any other serious condition.

Yoga can benefit people of any age, from children to older adults. Children take naturally to yoga and usually find it fun. Getting the whole family involved is one way to maintain the routine. Some adults find yoga complements their aerobic routine, while others engage in yoga as a great nonaerobic conditioner. It is possible to learn yoga from books or video tapes, but it is easier to learn from a teacher. Yoga classes are available in many places such as health clubs, community centers, universities, and hospitals.

Consistent practice of yoga will change your attitude about your body and your beliefs about what you can do to take care of yourself, both of which are crucial to well-being. For some, the physical exercise may be a way to attain a specific goal such as improving flexibility, improving muscle tone, or losing weight. Others have no specific goal other than the exercise itself and becoming aware of their self, breath, and energy. The relaxation that accompanies yoga can stimulate self-healing and contribute to a sense of inner peace.

Developing a Regular Yoga Practice

Benefits from any fitness program, including yoga, can occur only with continued practice. Try some of these suggestions to help develop a regular pattern:

- Make time for your practice every day; give yourself permission to take care of yourself and take time to relax. You may find that doing a few poses before bedtime or early in the morning works best. Even if you practice for only five minutes, a daily practice is the foundation on which to build.

- Many people find it helps to go to a yoga class at least once a week. The support of practicing with others and the information they get from teachers helps strengthen their commitment to yoga.

- You may want to create a dedicated yoga space. Temporarily push things aside to have enough space for your practice, or simply choose a place to spread your yoga mat on the floor. Having a regular space for practice will help you focus on the poses without distraction from your surroundings.

- Start with the poses you like. You might take one pose you like from each class and practice it at least once a day, which takes only a few moments. Gradually you can begin to combine the poses to form your own yoga session.

As you learn yoga, you will find that each sequence of poses will help you focus on something specific; for example, one sequence can improve balance, while another may release anger and negative feelings; some sequences will tone internal organs, increase lung capacity, or build upper-body strength. Choose the sequences that feel right for you. It is most important to remember that it is not a matter of being a beginning, intermediate, or advanced student but rather that you are a practicing student, doing as much as you can whenever you can. Yoga moves at your pace, in the time you have.

FIGURE 15.1

The Mountain Pose (*Tadasana*).

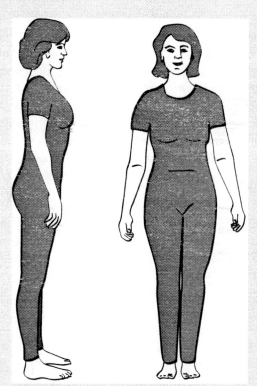

TRY IT YOURSELF: THE MOUNTAIN POSE *(TADASANA)*

Almost anyone can learn and benefit from the Mountain Pose, which is a standing position of postural awareness. When this pose is practiced well, the body is prepared for almost all daily movement: standing, sitting, walking, and running. Like the mountain poised between heaven and earth, this pose establishes grounding through the legs and feet and encourages the lift of the spine. Practice this while standing sideways near a full-length mirror at first so you can check your alignment (see Figure 15.1).

- Stand as shown in the diagram, with your feet close together, your knees straight, your shoulders back, and your head centered over your legs.

- Imagine your spinal column rising up tall and solid as a mountain, with your body balanced around it. Stretch your neck up and lift the back of your skull to further extend your spine.

- Hold your arms relaxed at your sides, palms toward your thighs. Lock your knees and raise your kneecaps. Relax your shoulders back and lift the collarbone.

- Breathe slowly and deeply, feeling the energy of the earth pour upwards into and through your body. Relax your face, look straight ahead, and hold the pose for 30 to 40 seconds, breathing evenly.

Practice the Mountain Pose several times a day. Standing well reduces strain on the joints, ligaments, and muscles, especially on those of the spinal column and lower extremities. It also aids respiration, digestion, and elimination, and conveys a sense of poise and self-esteem.

TRY IT YOURSELF: HEART BREATHING

1. Sit comfortably and close your eyes.

2. Simply notice your breathing without trying to change it. Pay attention to your in-breath and your out-breath.

3. Now imagine that the breath is pouring into your heart with each inhalation and flowing out of your heart with each exhalation. Just feel the breath flowing in and out of your heart. Imagine the breath is pure love.

4. Do this breath awareness for 5–10 minutes.

5. Now let your attention return to your environment, slowly open your eyes, get up, and move on.

6. Think about the feeling throughout the day.

A Yogic Pregnancy

One of many applications of yoga is in pregnancy and childbirth. In fact, many of the techniques taught in childbirth classes, such as focus, relaxation, and systematic breathing have their roots in yoga. The gentle stretching of the poses helps ease the muscle aches of pregnancy and strengthens the muscles that will be used during delivery. The breathing techniques may lessen the shortness of breath that often accompanies advanced pregnancy.

Yoga practiced while pregnant is slightly different from regular yoga in that some poses should not be attempted. These poses are the extreme stretching positions and any position that puts pressure on the uterus. Full forward bends will probably be uncomfortable for both woman and baby. Remember that your center of balance has shifted completely, and thus you must be careful with balance poses.

With midwife or doctor approval, most women can usually start gentle yoga poses two weeks after delivery, a few weeks longer if they have had a cesarean section.

caution

Pregnant women should never lie on the stomach for any pose. After the twentieth week, you should lie on their left side rather than your back. If any pose feels uncomfortable, stop at once. If you experience dizziness, sudden swelling, extreme shortness of breath, or vaginal bleeding, see a midwife or doctor immediately.

Start with a few poses and gradually work back to your regular routine. If postpartum bleeding gets heavier or brighter red, stop and call the midwife or doctor. Filling your body with energy through breathing exercises may promote self-healing after childbirth.

THE ABSOLUTE MINIMUM

- Yoga is an Indian system of health, postures, and living that aims to produce in its practitioners a state of perfect health and bliss.

- Most of the Western practice of yoga focuses on the physical exercises and postures, which promotes the flow of blood and energy through the body and can promote deep relaxation and health.

- A yoga practice can begin with matters as seemingly simple as breathing and standing, and can deepen into a full awareness of one's body, self, and place in the universe.

RESOURCES

- *Yoga Journal Magazine*

  www.yogajournal.com

- American Yoga Association

  www.americanyogaassociation.org/

- Bikram's Yoga College of India

  www.bikramyoga.com

- The Yoga Site

  www.yogasite.com

- *Light on Yoga*

  B.K.S. Iyengar, 1994, Schocken Books, New York

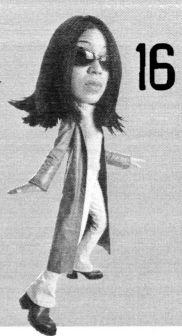

16

MEDITATION

Meditation is a general term for a wide range of practices that involve relaxing the body and stilling the mind. The latin root, *meditari*, means to consider, or to pay attention to something. As Dr. Jon Kabat-Zinn, the founder and director of the Stress Reduction Clinic at the University of Massachusetts Medical Center, states, "Meditation is simply about being yourself and knowing something about who that is. It is about coming to realize that you are on a path whether you like it or not—namely, the path that is your life. Meditation is the process by which we go about deepening our attention and awareness, refining them, and putting them to greater practical use in our lives."

The components of meditation are quite simple: a quiet space, a comfortable position, a receptive attitude, and a focus of attention. The relaxation response involves physiological and psychological effects that appear common to many forms of focused attention in addition to meditation: prayer, yoga, biofeedback, and the pre-suggestion phase of hypnosis. Meditation is a process that anyone can use to calm down, cope with stress, and, for those with spiritual inclinations, feel as one with God or the universe. Meditation can be practiced individually or in groups and is easy to learn. It requires no change in belief system and is compatible with most religious practices.

What Is Meditation?

Most meditative practices have come to the West from Eastern practices, particularly those of India, China, Japan, and Tibet. Meditative techniques, however, can be found in most cultures of the world where prayer, meditation, ritual, or contemplation are all initiated by shifting into a relaxed state. Nearly all major religions include some form of meditative practice. Christianity, Judaism, Buddhism, and Islam all use repetitive prayers, chants, or movements as part of their worship rituals. Although religious practices in the West are not typically labeled "meditative," they in fact are. The Catholic practice of using rosary beads while saying the "Hail Mary" is a familiar example. The repetition of the words combined with the movement of the beads induces a state of relaxation and a quieting of the mind.

Until recently, the primary purpose of meditation has been spiritual or religious. Since the 1970s, it has been explored as a way of reducing stress on both body and mind. Many conventional healthcare practitioners recommend it for widely diverse situations from natural childbirth to managing hypertension to pain control. For many years, nurses have taught clients progressive relaxation in a wide variety of clinical settings.

Practicing meditation does not require a teacher and many people learn the process through instruction from books or audiotapes. Some people, however, find that the structure of a meditation class is helpful. Many varieties of teachers and classes are available. Currently no certification process is available for a meditation teacher. The general standard is some years of daily meditation practice before one teaches others. Both Christian and Buddhist traditions offer regular classes and retreats designed to teach meditative practices and the process of being a spiritual being in a material world. In the Hindu tradition, people learn meditation from a guru who is a spiritual teacher or guide. Whatever the tradition, teachers encourage self-responsibility and the practice of mindfulness in everyday life.

How Does Meditation Work?

Meditation is both simple and difficult: simple because it is nothing more than maintaining focused attention, difficult because of the habitual, lifelong pattern of letting the mind wander wherever it wants. With extended practice, the mind tends to become better and better at staying focused. The stability and calmness that come with focused attention are the foundation of meditation.

Meditative State

Meditation is about being aware of who one is in the here-and-now rather than about feeling a particular way. It means letting go of any expectations of the process and simply observing what happens as it unfolds. People are sometimes concerned that they do not have the skills to meditate. As Dr. Kabat-Zinn states, "Thinking you are unable to meditate is a little like thinking you are unable to breathe, or to concentrate or relax. Pretty much everybody can breathe easily. And under the right circumstances, pretty much anybody can concentrate, anybody can relax." All forms of meditation require regular, daily practice over a period of time to experience the many benefits.

Attention and Concentration

Basic to all meditative techniques is the intentional focus of attention on one thought, word, sound, image, or physical sensation for a sustained period of time. The mind is fully alert but not focused on the external world or events. The normal rapid series of thoughts and feelings are replaced with inner awareness and attention. Rather than the mind jumping around between the past and the future, attention is in the present reality. It is impossible to make the mind empty, but it is possible to focus on one thing which helps the mind let go of the tendency to worry, plan, think, analyze, remember, or solve problems. A passive, nonjudgmental attitude is necessary during meditation. When thoughts intrude, they are noticed, and then let go as the attention returns to the original focus.

In some types of meditation, the focus is on the breath, the primary purpose being to calm the mind and body. It is a process of keeping the attention on the breath while breathing deeply, slowly, and regularly. The awareness is on the breath moving in and the breath moving out, and allowing all other thoughts, feelings, or sensations to pass by as this focus is maintained. Through regular meditation practice, it becomes a habit to breathe more consciously and deeply throughout the day, so that in the long run, the breath becomes a calming force in daily life.

Focal Points for the Empty Mind

Some people use a mantra as their focus of attention. A *mantra* is a sound or sounds that resonate in the body and evoke certain energies. Mantras, such as OM, soothe the mind and awaken the senses. Another beginning mantra is OM SHANTI SHANTI SHANTI. *Shanti* means peace, and when repeated three times, it balances the body, mind, and spirit.

A mandala meditation uses an object to focus the mind through sight. A *mandala* is a circular geometric design that draws the eye to the center and is meant to suggest the universe's circular patterns from atoms to solar systems. Mandalas appear as labyrinths in the floors of some cathedrals in Europe. The faithful follow the course of the labyrinth into the center as penitence or in spiritual contemplation. Mandalas have recently become popular in the United States among some Christian religious groups who are renewing the contemplative aspects of their faith (see Figure 16.1). Using mantras and mandalas together is an effective focus for meditation.

FIGURE 16.1

The Walking Mandala from the Cathedral at Chartres.

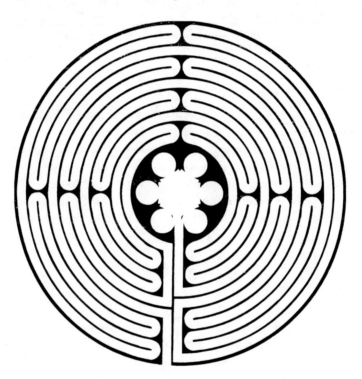

Better Living Through Less Stress

Many disorders or diseases are aggravated or caused by stress, which overstimulates the limbic systems of the brain, which controls our moods, sleep cycles, libido, and emotions. In addition, overactivity of the sympathetic nervous system and exhaustion of the adrenal glands are related to stress. It is thought that excessive limbic activity may inhibit immune function, which may account for the association of chronic stress and increased susceptibility to infection.

A relaxed state is the opposite of the aroused state of fight or flight. The fight-or-flight reflex increases blood pressure, heart rate, breathing, metabolism, and blood flow to the muscles. The response triggered by all the relaxing practices does the opposite and results in a lower blood pressure and slower heart rate, breathing, metabolism, and blood flow. Relaxation and meditation also decrease the production of neurotransmitters like dopamine and epinephrine, thereby decreasing limbic activity. Since the state of mind, the emotional, attitudinal, and intellectual components of oneself, initiates activities in the nervous system, people can consciously choose to trigger the benefits of meditation. Some relief can be found from simply taking a deep breath, relaxing, and repeating the words: "My body, mind, and spirit are always working to keep me supremely well."

Meditation techniques offer the potential of learning how to live in an increasingly complex and stressful society while helping to preserve health in the process. Given their low cost and demonstrated health benefits, these simple mental technologies may be some of the best candidates among the alternative therapies for widespread inclusion in medical practice and for investment of medical resources.

Achieving the Relaxation Response

The relaxation response can be evoked by any number of techniques, including progressive relaxation, meditation, prayer, jogging, swimming, Lamaze breathing exercises, yoga, T'ai Chi, and Qigong. The beauty of these techniques is their simplicity. They allow the mind to have a focus while enhancing one's vitality and well-being.

The varieties of meditation have many different names. Some are religious practices and some are not. Some are complicated while some are simple. Each type of meditative practice involves a form of mental focusing and the adoption of a nonjudgmental attitude toward intruding thoughts. All types appear to produce similar physical and psychological changes. People beginning the practice of meditation should look around for a type of meditation that seems comfortable, that involves a technique they can follow, and that does not conflict with their belief system.

Transcendental Meditation

Transcendental Meditation (TM) was developed by the Indian leader Maharishi Mahesh Yogi in an effort to make the ancient practice of meditation more attainable to Westerners. TM is a sound-focused form of meditation and is simple and easy to learn. To prevent distracting thoughts, a person is given a mantra (a word or sound) to repeat silently over and over again while sitting in a comfortable position. When thoughts other than the mantra come to mind, the person is to notice them, and then gently return the focus to the mantra. It is expected that people will practice TM for 20 minutes, once or twice a day. The trademarked Transcendental Meditation is a commercial enterprise that is a fairly expensive undertaking. Classes are typically found in Ayurveda schools and healthcare centers. Local centers may be found on the Internet at www.tm.org.

Buddhist Meditation

The essence of Buddhist meditation is training the mind in compassion and in wisdom. The goal is to develop compassion for all living things. Meditation begins with a time of contemplation, which typically includes the following points:

- Just as I wish to be free from suffering and experience only happiness, so do all other beings.
- I am no different from any other being; we are all equal.
- My happiness and suffering are insignificant when compared with the happiness and suffering of all other living beings.

The next step in the meditation process is meditating on any determinations that might have been made during contemplation. Your meditative practice concludes by dedicating your life and purpose to the welfare of all living beings. It is believed that many of the daily problems people experience will disappear, because most of them arise from regarding yourself as more important than others.

Mindfulness

Mindfulness, an ancient Buddhist practice, is both a philosophy as well as a meditation practice. Its primary principle is "being in the moment." Most people go through daily routines with little awareness or attention.

People read while they eat, exercise while watching TV, or cook while talking to their children, and the nuances of these experiences are lost. This situation might be called living mindlessly by ignoring present moments. Mindfulness is the opposite of living on "automatic pilot." It is the art of conscious living through focusing full attention on the activity at hand. While it may be simple to practice mindfulness, it is not necessarily easy. Habitual unawareness is persistent and mindfulness requires effort and discipline. Thus, to eat a peach mindfully would involve being actively aware of every sensation, every smell, every taste, noticing its texture, its color, its weight, and how it feels on the tongue. This technique can be practiced with any activity.

Mindfulness meditation is a daily practice that encourages living in the moment. It begins by sitting quietly with your eyes closed and focusing on your breathing. The flow of thought during the meditation is observed as thoughts come and go. The key to mindfulness meditation is the ability to accept rather than judge the wandering thoughts, bringing attention back to the breathing as needed.

Tibetan Meditation

Tibetan meditation is a breath-focused form of meditation. You simply focus attention on each in-breath and out-breath. When thoughts about anything other than the breath intrude, you note them by silently saying "thinking," and then attention is returned to the breath. It is recognized that thought cannot be completely halted and that thoughts are a natural process and are simply to be noted in a nonjudgmental way.

Moving Meditation

Forms of moving meditation include the Chinese martial art T'ai Chi, the Japanese martial art Aikido, the Indian practice of yoga, and the walking meditation in Zen Buddhism. Instead of focusing on a word or on breathing, movement meditations use physical sensations as the focus of concentration. In walking meditation, for example, attention is given to the feeling of each step as it is taken. Intruding thoughts are simply noticed and attention is returned to the step. Research has found that focused walking, in contrast to unfocused walking, is associated with reduced anxiety and fewer negative thoughts.

How Do I Start a Meditation Practice?

If practiced regularly, even 15 minutes twice a day, meditation produces widespread positive effects on physical and psychological functioning. The autonomic nervous system responds with a decrease in heart rate, lower blood pressure, decreased respiratory rate and oxygen consumption, and a lower arousal threshold.

Why Meditate?

People who meditate say that they have clearer minds and sharper thoughts. The brain seems to clear itself so that new ideas and beliefs become available. This clearer mind may be accompanied by a cognitive restructuring in which people interpret life events in a more positive, more realistic fashion. Meditation's residual effects—improved stress-coping abilities—are a protection against daily stress and anxiety. All other self-healing methods are improved with the practice of meditation.

Some adverse effects of meditation are possible. Relaxation exercises should not be practiced while driving or operating potentially dangerous machinery. Some people have been stressed so long that they are unfamiliar with deep relaxation and therefore feel threatened by it. In meditation, people are taught to accept nonjudgmentally whatever thoughts occur. Sometimes, however, extremely upsetting thoughts arise and it is impossible to remain nonjudgmental, which could lead to disparaging thoughts about one's abilities. The adverse effects for more experienced meditators are temporary fear, anxiety, confusion, depression, or self-doubt. For an unknown reason, these kinds of thoughts are more likely to arise during the first 10 minutes of meditation. In rare instances, relaxation exercises may trigger seizures in people with sleep onset seizure disorders. People with schizophrenia may experience an acute episode following intensive meditation. Meditation may also be inappropriate for people with extreme anger, hostility, or obsessive thoughts, because they may be unable to quiet their minds adequately and therefore may not perceive the experience as relaxing.

Beginning Your Practice

A meditative practice consists of two basic activities:

- The repetition of a word, sound, prayer, phrase, idea, or muscular activity
- The disregard of everyday thoughts that interfere with the process.

The sidebar lists focus words or prayers that you may find appropriate. The word or phrase is silently repeated with each in-breath and out-breath. Some people choose to use one word for the in-breath and another for the out-breath. Some meditators choose an object of personal significance on which to focus. Every detail of the object is studied, including gradations of shape, color, texture, and so on. Flowers, candle flames, or religious statues are common choices.

MEDITATION FOCUS WORDS

SECULAR FOCUS WORDS

One

Ocean

Love

Peace

Well-being

Let it be

Relax

RELIGIOUS FOCUS WORDS OR PRAYERS

CHRISTIAN

"Our Father who art in heaven"

"The Lord is my shepherd"

"Hail, Mary, full of grace"

"Lord Jesus Christ have mercy on me"

JEWISH

"Sh'ma Yisroel"

"Shalom"

"Echod"

"The Lord is my shepherd"

ISLAMIC

"Insha'allah"

HINDU

"Om"

Before sitting down to meditate, it is helpful to make sure that the area is clean and uncluttered, which helps keep the mind clear and fresh. No props are required for meditation, although some people may choose to include incense, candles, or religious symbols in their meditative practice. Beginners often start with 5–10 minutes of meditation and increase the time gradually. It is most important that time is scheduled each day, and many people find that meditating first thing in the morning, before the busy day begins, works well. Other people prefer to meditate in the evening. The key is to find a time when one is unlikely to be disturbed. It is best to wait about two hours after a big meal, during which time the blood flow is diverted from the brain to the gut.

PROGRESSIVE RELAXATION

Progressive relaxation is a way of decreasing muscular tension in about 10 minutes. It should be done in a quiet place, in any comfortable position, although typically it is done lying on your back. Begin by focusing on your breath, breathing gently, slowly, and deeply. Shift your awareness different parts of the body in turn, by tensing a muscle groups as tight as possible, holding the tension for several seconds, and then consciously relaxing it. Start with your toes and slowly work up the body, tensing your feet, calves, thighs, butt, abdomen, chest arms, neck and face. Experience the difference between a muscle that is tense and one that is relaxed.

THE BODY SCAN MEDITATION

- Lie on your back with your legs uncrossed, your arms at your sides, palms up, and your eyes closed.

- Focus on your breathing, breathing in peace and breathing out tension.

- As you begin to feel relaxed, direct your attention to your feet, paying attention to any sensations. Let your feet relax and feel the warmth spread throughout your feet.

- Then move your focus to your ankles. Follow the same procedure as you move up your lower legs, knees, thighs, hips, and so on all around the body.

- Pay particular attention to any areas that are painful or are the focus of any medical condition such as the lungs or heart.

- Finish the body scan by paying particular attention to the neck and head. Experience the warmth of the relaxation.

All sitting meditative practices begin with finding a comfortable but erect position. The posture itself is a meditation. Slumping reflects low energy and passivity, while a ramrod-straight posture reflects tension and effort. It is easiest to meditate if the spine is straight and the body posture is symmetrical. Some people sit on the floor cross-legged using a firm cushion under their backside to support the spine. Others sit in a chair with a straight back, with both feet on the ground. The face relaxes, shoulders drop, and head, neck, and back move into easy alignment. The eyes may be either open or closed. Hands may be resting in the lap or may be held with palms together. It is believed that having the palms together with the fingertips touching completes a circuit of energy extending from the heart down the arms and through the chakras in the center of the palm of each hand as well as the chakras in the fingertips. People often experiment with various ways of positioning their hands during meditation until they find what is best for them.

TRY IT YOURSELF: A GENERAL-PURPOSE MEDITATION PROCESS

The following process may be useful when starting your meditation practice. You should feel free to modify it as you discover what works best for you:

1. Pick a focus word or short phrase that is firmly rooted in your belief system.

2. Sit quietly in a comfortable position.

3. Close your eyes.

4. Relax your muscles.

5. Breathe slowly and naturally, and as you do, repeat your focus word, phrase, or prayer silently to yourself as you exhale.

6. Assume a passive attitude. Don't worry about how well you're doing. When other thoughts come to mind, simply say to yourself, "Oh, well," and gently return to the repetition.

7. Continue for 10–20 minutes.

8. Do not stand immediately. Continue sitting quietly for a minute or so, allowing other thoughts to return. Then open your eyes and sit for another minute before rising.

9. Practice this technique once or twice daily.

Enriching and Extending Your Meditative Practice

One type of meditation is an awareness of breathing meditation. Concentrate on the sensation of the breath as it enters your nose and fills your chest and abdomen, and again as it passes out of your body. Alternatively, one can imagine the breath coming in from the toes, up the legs, through the belly, and into the chest and out the same pathway. It is helpful to imagine healing and relaxation flowing into the body with each in-breath, and stress or pain leaving the body with each out-breath. When thoughts arise, they are noticed, and then let go as attention is brought back to the breathing.

Another awareness of breathing practice is a simple technique used in Zen meditation. Sit in a comfortable position with the spine straight, gently close your eyes and breathe naturally and easily. To begin the exercise, count "one" to yourself as you exhale. On the next exhale, count "two," and so on up to "five." Then begin a new cycle, counting "one" on the next exhale. Never count higher than "five" and count only on when you exhale. You will know your attention has wandered when you find yourself counting "eight" or "ten." When this occurs, gently refocus and restart on the count of "one." This form of meditation should be done for about ten minutes.

Any repetitive behavior can be used as a meditative focus. One of the most universally used practices is walking meditation. In walking meditation, you are not walking to get anyplace. Having no place to go makes it easier to be where you are. It is often done some place in nature, on a track, on a walking mandala, or even pushing a shopping cart through a supermarket. It can be practiced at any pace, from very slow to very brisk. In practice, you take each step as it comes and you are fully present with it. You notice the movements of each foot, how it lifts, moves forward in space, and then descends again. Just as in other forms of meditation, when you begin to think, the thoughts are let go and awareness is returned to the physical sensations of walking.

There are as many ways to meditate as there are people. When people say they have tried meditation and cannot do it, they just have not found the right practice for them. You may want to sit, do repetitive prayers, swim or run, walk, or do yoga or T'ai Chi. Explore a variety of techniques and develop the habit of meditation on a daily basis.

The Absolute Minimum

- Meditation is a process of stilling the mind and deepening your internal awareness.

- Meditation can bring deep relaxation, with a reduction in stress and its health-related side effects.

- There are as many ways to meditate as there are minds to still; everyone can meditate and find a practice that works for them.

Resources

- American Meditation Institute

  www.americanmeditation.org

- The World Wide Online Meditation Center

  www.meditationcenter.com

- Books

  Lawrence Leshan, *How to Meditate*, Little, Brown & Company, 1999

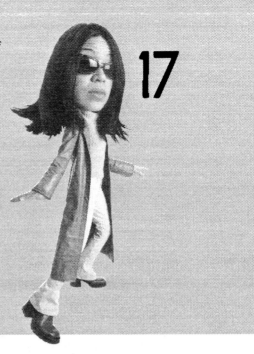

17

HYPNOTHERAPY

Hypnotherapy is the application of hypnosis in a wide variety of medical and psychological disorders. Hypnosis is a state of attentive and focused concentration during which people are highly responsive to suggestion. Guided imagery, in a state of focused concentration, is a similar process that encourages changes in attitudes, behavior, and physiological reactions. Many people consider guided imagery to be a form of hypnosis.

Hypnotherapists and guided imagery therapists help people learn methods to take advantage of the mind/body/spirit connection through the medium of relaxation and imagination. The basic difference between meditation and hypnosis, or guided imagery, is that in meditation you empty your mind of images, while in hypnosis or guided imagery, you create vivid mental images.

What Is Hypnotherapy?

Around the world, shamans and traditional healers have used the power of suggested mental images for thousands of years. Hypnotic trances were used in a variety of healing practices and religious rituals such as holding sweat lodge ceremonies, drumming, and chanting. Inducing trance states and using therapeutic suggestion were central practices of the early Greek healing temples. People in the 14th century thought illness was related to evil spirits, and evil spirits were often treated with imagery and hypnotic techniques. During the Renaissance (14th–16th centuries), it was believed that dysfunctional imagination was the root of all pathology. It was even believed that the mother's imaginings during pregnancy could alter the growth and development of her child.

Hypnotherapy began in the late 18th century in Europe with an Austrian physician, Franz Anton Mesmer, who is considered the father of hypnosis. He is remembered for the term *mesmerize*, which described a process of inducing trance through a series of passes he made with his hands and/or magnets over people. He worked with psychic and electromagnetic energies that he called animal magnetism. The medical community eventually discredited him despite his considerable success treating a variety of ailments. In the mid-19th century, James Braid, an English physician, successfully used hypnosis in pain control and as an anesthetic in surgery. Even after witnessing live demonstrations of a patient undergoing painless surgery, his colleagues dismissed him as a fake. Not long afterward, the discovery of chloroform led to the near abandonment of hypnotic anesthesia.

In the late 19th and early 20th centuries, Emile Coue, a French physician, formulated the Laws of Suggestion, discussed later in this chapter and used to this day by hypnotherapists. He also discovered that giving positive suggestions when prescribing medication proved to be a more effective cure than prescribing medication alone. Sigmund Freud at first found hypnosis extremely effective in treating hysteria, and then, troubled by the sudden emergence of powerful emotions in his patients, he abandoned it in favor of psychoanalysis. Carl Jung did not actively use hypnosis, but he encouraged his patients to use active imagination to change old memories. He often used the concept of the inner guide in his healing work. Milton Erickson, an American psychologist and psychiatrist, is considered the father of modern hypnotherapy. He demonstrated how traumatic amnesia and psychosomatic symptoms can be resolved with hypnotherapy and was influential in the official acceptance of hypnotherapy by the American Medical Association in 1958.

While anyone can hypnotize other people, it is best for hypnotherapy to be administered by healthcare professionals. At present, no laws limit the use of hypnosis to clinical practitioners. However, nurses, physicians, dentists, psychologists, social workers, and counselors are eligible to take approved professional training in hypnotherapy. The American Society of Clinical Hypnosis (ASCH) and The Society for Clinical and Experimental Hypnosis (SCEH) share in the education and accrediting of people who meet professional requirements. Most practitioners do not identify themselves as hypnotists but as nurses, doctors, dentists, and others who use hypnosis as one of several modes of intervention.

The Nature of Hypnotherapy

To understand hypnosis, one must understand the functional difference between the conscious and subconscious mind. The conscious mind contains the short-term memory and the intellect. It functions like a computer, always analyzing, criticizing, and discriminating one's thoughts and perceptions. The language of the intellect is logic and reason. The subconscious mind contains emotions, creativity, imagination, intuition, long-term memory, and control of bodily functions. It also contains the habit center where persistent habits such as nail biting or test anxiety are located. The subconscious does not respond to reason and facts, as does the intellect. The language of the subconscious is imagery and metaphor. During times of emotional turmoil or sudden trauma, people often become aware of the subconscious mind's power over bodily functions and intellect when they are unable to eat, sleep, or talk, and cannot think clearly. After years of ignoring feelings or "stuffing" them into the subconscious, in a hypnotic trance, people can access their subconscious mind, which allows them to tap into their creativity, access buried memories, change habits, unmask erroneous beliefs, repair self-esteem, and restore health.

Trance: Letting the Subconscious Drive

A trance state is a form of heightened concentration. People in trances are aware of what is going on around them but choose not to focus on it and can return to normal awareness whenever they choose. The majority of people will tend to remember most of what happens in a controlled hypnotherapy or guided imagery session. Trance is not a form of sleep or stupor, as is easily determined by observing the range of activities possible by people in a hypnotic trance.

People naturally flow in and out of hypnotic trances. When driving a familiar route, people may slip into a trance. They arrive at their destination, not sure exactly how they got there. During the trance they drive appropriately, stop at stop signs, obey traffic laws, and so on, but have no conscious awareness of doing these things. Another example of hypnotic trance occurs during movies. People enter the theater having set aside a specific period of time wherein they can enjoy themselves. The process of settling into theater seats relaxes moviegoers and puts them in a receptive frame of mind. The lights go down to reduce the distractions from the outside world and the big screen becomes the most noticeable aspect of one's perceptual world. Within moments, the audience is transported to another place and time. If the movie is frightening, many people experience a racing heart, rapid breathing, and muscle tension—yet they are well aware that no physical danger exists. They are responding to images and sounds alone. Movies work by similar mental mechanisms as hypnosis. First participants decide to let go of normal concerns and open the mind to a new experience. Then certain procedures relax the beta level of brain activity. Then, through the thoughtful use of metaphor and imagery, deeper levels of consciousness are reached. Finally, new images and perceptions can be introduced.

A trance is characterized by muscle relaxation, predominating alpha brain waves, feelings of well-being, diminished ability to vocalize, and an ability to accept new ideas if not in conflict with personal values. The perception of time is often distorted; thirty minutes may seem like five minutes. Feelings are more accessible while entranced, as well as memories from long ago. As one's awareness phases in and out, parts of the session may not be consciously remembered but are retained in the subconscious. People in trance describe their arms and legs as feeling heavy like lead or light and tingly, almost numb. Some experience slight twitches as the nervous system relaxes, and respiration shifts to abdominal breathing. Coming out of the trance, people awaken with very pleasant, almost euphoric feelings of well-being.

Bark Like a Dog: Laws and Principles of Suggestion

The first law of suggestion, as formulated by Coue, is that of concentrated attention. When people focus their attention repeatedly on a goal or idea, that event tends to be realized. Based on this belief, practitioners repeat hypnotic suggestions three or four times during a session. The law of dominant effect states that stronger emotions tend to take precedence over weaker ones. An effective hypnotherapist, after assessing the client's emotional state, connects the hypnotic suggestion to the dominant emotions. The carrot principle is applied when the practitioner interjects comments about the person's goals with the hypnotic suggestions, thus linking motivation to the suggestions. The principle of positive suggestion is applied to help people override existing attitudes. Dr. Coue was known for encouraging his patients to say to themselves 20–30 times each night before going to sleep, "Everyday in every way, I am getting better and better." If someone is seeking hypnosis in an effort to lose weight, the positive suggestion is not, "You will not be hungry," which is unlikely and a negative rather than positive statement. Rather the positive suggestion might be, "You will be surprised to find how comfortable you will be. Treat your body with kindness and respect."

Memories

It is true that under hypnosis people often recall past forgotten events. It is also true that people under hypnosis often "remember" things quite vividly that never actually happened, but which have great personal significance nonetheless. These might be called fantasized life events. In a deep trance state, memories and fantasies may be intense, and the two may be indistinguishable. People are able to remember great detail of actual events and are also uniquely capable of making up details and experiencing them as if they were remembered. Recognizing the potential difficulties arising from what some call "false memory syndrome," several states in the United States now limit legal testimony to that obtained prior to any systematic hypnotic treatment. In 1985, the American Medical Association cautioned against the systematic use of hypnosis for memory recall for both its unreliability and its potential to create vivid false memories.

You Are Feeling Sleepy, Very Sleepy: The Process of Hypnosis

Hypnotherapists do not "put" people into trances. They arrange circumstances to increase the likelihood that people will shift themselves into a trance state. About 20% of the population has a high capacity for trance; these people may go under hypnosis deeply. Another 20% has a slight capacity for trance, are easily distracted, and may not respond to hypnotherapy at all. People who cannot be hypnotized include those with organic brain disease, those with low IQ, and those who do not want to be hypnotized. The remaining 60% falls somewhere between these extremes.

For people seeking hypnotherapy or guided imagery, the question arises as to whether the use of audio tapes would offer equal benefit. The answer to that question depends on several factors, including the nature and depth of the problem to resolve. General self-hypnosis tapes will give only general results. Personalized audio tapes, created by a therapist using the individual's own images, are more effective. Working with an experienced practitioner is most effective because the procedure is individualized according to the client's expectations and preferences.

Establishing a Healing Relationship

The first and most important step in hypnotherapy is establishing a relationship with the client. It is a cooperative venture, and if the suggestions are to be effective, the therapist and client must work together. The relationship is one in which clients are as receptive as possible, and the therapist commits to working for the clients' well-being. The therapist gets to know clients, develops treatment plans, explains the hypnotic process, dispels myths and fears, answers questions, encourages positive attitudes about hypnosis, and with people's permission, trains them in self-inductive procedures. This process is as applicable for a short-term case of test anxiety as it is for a lengthy terminal illness. A measure of trust is needed to start the process and to develop the relationship.

Entering the Subconscious

The induction phase is generally a period of relaxation or focus on the breathing that disengages people from other concerns and helps them focus their attention. In other words, the induction phase is similar to meditation and elicits the same physiological response. The induction starts with "easy" suggestions, such as focusing on breathing and closing the eyes. Directions are given to relax physically and mentally and to focus on the therapist's voice and words.

Training in induction may take one or two sessions. When the client is comfortable with entering the trance experience, the hypnotic suggestion begins. Based on the assessment process, the practitioner suggests an image known to be pleasurable to the client and related to the desired outcome. Hypnotic communications contain cues and explicit instructions for focusing attention and imagining in line with the aims of suggestions.

Making the Suggestion

The imagery is intensified by incorporating the five senses: The person is asked not only to visualize the scene but to smell the scents, touch things in the environment, hear the surrounding sounds, and even taste anything appropriate. The client is asked to focus attention on as many details about the situation as possible, and then is walked through the session focusing on the desired events. The hypnotherapist's suggestions of are translated by the client into ideas. These ideas then lead to corresponding behaviors in the nontrance state.

When the directions of the hypnotherapist help the patient imagine a situation when the desired change has already been made, the process is sometimes referred to as Guided Imagery (GI), which is explored in more detail later in the chapter.

Snapping the Fingers

Trance removal is when clients are given suggestions that return them to a non-trance state. The hypnotherapist, for example, may count to 10, asking clients to open their eyes at the count of 5, and to be fully alert at 10. Clients most commonly report that they feel relaxed during the session but may not be certain that they were hypnotized, since they could hear every word the therapist said. Many hypnotherapists provide guided audio tapes for their clients so they can practice the therapy at home.

Hypnosis cannot make people do anything against their will. If they really do not want to change, hypnosis will be a waste of time and money. If, for example, a person seeks hypnotherapy to stop smoking at a spouse's insistence but is poorly motivated, hypnotherapy will not be effective. Occasionally clients may demand that the hypnotherapist perform some magical incantation and remove 30 pounds or make the person never smoke again. This demand is the equivalent of insisting that their primary care provider cure them of hypertension while refusing to change their diet or follow a recommended medication schedule.

In some medical facilities, hypnosis and imagery are now routinely used with a variety of conditions, usually in conjunction with other forms of medical, surgical, psychiatric, or psychological treatment. Hypnosis and imagery can be used with nonmedical clients as well, who want to work through problems of living, situations of performance anxiety, and in changing bad habits. Depending on the complexity and seriousness of the complaint, treatment typically runs from 2 to 10 sessions.

Benefits and Applications of Hypnotherapy

Hypnotherapy and guided imagery can be used to help gain self-control, improve self-esteem, and become more autonomous. People who are imprisoned by negative beliefs see themselves as hopeless, helpless victims. With guided imagery, they can learn how to substitute positive, empowering messages. Hypnosis and imagery also can be used as a mental rehearsal for procedures, treatments, or surgery. Clients are shown how to use their own images about the healing process or, alternatively, they are guided through a series of images that are intended to distract them from painful procedures or anxiety-producing situations. The practitioner may have clients imagine themselves in a state of good health, well-being, or successfully achieved goals.

People, especially children, are often able to rid themselves of warts by visualizing their disappearance in one way or another. Hypnosis and imagery are often used as a clinical treatment for Reynaud's disease, a condition in which the capillaries of the extremities constrict, with the result that hands and feet are cold and painful. When they learn to "think warm," people may find that the circulation to their hands and feet improves, resulting in less pain.

Similarly, hand-warming frequently cuts down on both the incidence and severity of migraine headaches. The use of hypnosis in promoting feelings of comfort, distraction, and dissociation through imagery in those with chronic pain has been well established. Clients are often able to change their perceptual experience of pain by substituting numbness, a sense of pressure, or other sensation for an unwanted pain.

Much of the literature regarding the use of imagery for cancer is anecdotal but many people believe the reports must be respected. Jeanne Achterberg well known for her use of imagery in the treatment of cancer believes that imagery is as essential as radiation and chemotherapy and must not be thought of as a "last alternative." She believes that imagery plays an important role in the biochemical healing process. She believes that images produced in the mind are converted to biochemical messages that somehow initiate a path of cancer-cell destruction or organ-cell reconstruction. It is possible that this healing process inhibits the nervous and endocrine systems from secreting stress hormones. Of course, it is difficult to prove definitively that imagery is a direct cause of healing when it occurs, because imagery is never the sole treatment used.

EVIL GENIUSES, LOOK ELSEWHERE

Hypnosis and imagery will only work if you want them to. Poor motivation, such as "My husband sent me so I would lose weight," an unwillingness even to try the treatment because of extreme fear, or compelling religious objections will all preclude progress through hypnotherapy. The procedure is unsuitable for people with active psychosis or somatic delusions. It is generally considered that these individuals are often bombarded with too many images already, and are unable to differentiate between voluntary and involuntary images.

Guided Imagery

A subtype of hypnotherapy is Guided Imagery (GI). It involves making changes to the psyche by entering a hypnotic-like state and imagining that the desired change has already occurred. GI can be practiced with or without a hypnotherapist.

Feeling-State Imagery

Feeling-state imagery is designed to simply help people change their mood in a general way. You can let your imagination take you to a favorite place, real or imagined. For example, some may imagine themselves at a beach and floating gently on the water, while feeling peaceful and relaxed. Others may imagine themselves as a young child sitting on the lap of a beloved grandparent. Using this kind of imagery can help you move from a state of tension and fear to one of peace and calm.

End-State Imagery

End-state imagery occurs when patients imagine themselves already in the situation or circumstances that they desire. For example, seeing one's self as healthy, strong, and free from disease. Others may imagine themselves as successful, happy, and well loved.

Energetic Imagery

Symptoms of disease are often thought to result from blocked energy. Energetic imagery involves imagining the life force energy, or *qi*, flowing smoothly and easily throughout the body. Imagine that you are pulling up energy from the earth through the soles of your feet, replenishing your body's energy.

Cellular Imagery

Cellular imagery relates to imagining events at the cellular level. For example, you imagine your natural killer cells surrounding and attacking cancer cells. Cellular imagery is usually specific and focused on exactly what needs to be fixed. Imagery does not have to be visual. Some people "hear" their imagery, others "feel" it, and some "taste" or "smell" it. Some people might choose to put a hand over the affected area and send healing images to the cells in that area.

Psychological Imagery

Similar to cellular imagery, physiological imagery involves the entire body. You might imagine that your blood vessels are relaxed and wider in an effort to lower blood pressure. People with back pain may imagine that all the muscles in their back are relaxing and softening. People with diabetes may put their hands over the abdomen and imagine insulin moving out of the pancreas to connect with hungry cells throughout the body.

Psychological imagery involves people's perception of themselves. For example, people who feel overly responsible may feel as though they have the weight of the world on their shoulders. Those who feel abandoned may feel the pain as heartache. You may want to put your hands on the hurting places, and breathe into the pain. Psychological imagery can also be interactive. When conflict is the issue, you can imagine a dialogue with the adversary that may bring a fresh perspective and new solutions to problems.

Spiritual Imagery

The goal of spiritual imagery is to make contact with God or the Divine, gain entrance into a larger world, or find guidance or inspiration. Some people find it comforting to imagine that they are being held in the hands of God where they are perfectly safe.

How Do I Get Started with Hypnotherapy?

Some people fear that hypnosis and guided imagery may cause them to lose control of their minds to an outside force. The reality is quite the opposite because the individual is always under self-control. When clients learn a technique like imagery, it is entirely within their control, for use when, how, and where they want. It is a tool that can be used whenever a person feels particularly anxious, upset, or uncomfortable. That type of empowering, in itself, is healing, because people feel better and do better when they have a sense of mastery over what is happening to them.

TRY IT YOURSELF: SELF-HYPNOSIS TECHNIQUES

RENOVATING YOUR DAY

This exercise is designed to empower yourself with your thoughts by transforming negative thoughts and events through visualization. Do this every day for a week, prior to bedtime. Mentally go through your day and decide what you could have changed that would have brought better results. Then imagine that change happening. For example, if someone said something to you that you did not like, imagine something more positive was said. If you did not like your test score, visualize the grade as a better one.

SHRINKING ANTAGONISTIC FORCES

If you are angry with or intimidated by another person, shrink that person and put him/her in the palm of your open hand. Have a discussion with that person but have that person talk in a different voice, like a high, squeaky or cartoon voice. See that person getting smaller and smaller until the person disappears or you blow him/her off into space.

THE PINK BUBBLE: A GUIDED IMAGERY EXERCISE

The pink bubble technique can be done as a one-time experience or regularly over a period of time. It is best to do the technique in the morning when you first wake up and/or in the evening right before sleep. This technique works as follows:

- Assume a comfortable position, breathe slowly, and go through a progressive relaxation or body scan procedure.
- Imagine something you would like to have or would like to have happen.
- Imagine that it has already happened. Picture the object or the situation as clearly as possible, with yourself in the picture.
- Surround this image with a pink bubble.
- Let go of the bubble and watch the bubble float off into the universe. See it becoming one with the higher power of the universe.

THE ABSOLUTE MINIMUM

- Hypnotherapy can help patients access healing energies and experiences within their subconscious minds.
- With a willing and engaged patient, hypnotic suggestion can help break addictions and encourage healthy behavior.
- By combining guided imagery with hypnosis, patients can imagine healing taking place within themselves; the power of their minds makes the healing take place.

RESOURCES

- Academy for Guided Imagery

    www.interactiveimagery.com

- American Board of Hypnotherapy

    www.aih.cc

18

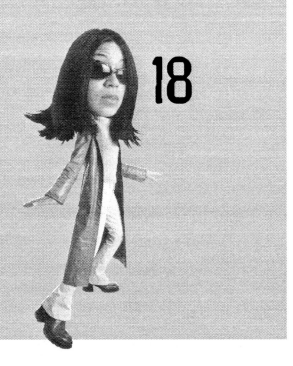

DREAMWORK

In some ways, a great deal is known about dreaming, because it has been important to people for all time and across all cultures. In the 20th century, the biology of the brain has been explored and increasingly understood. While this basic knowledge provides some facts underlying dreaming, it does not tell us what dreaming is. Thus, in a sense, little is known about dreaming, and scientists cannot yet agree on the basic nature of dreaming. Some believe dreams are nothing more than random firing of neurons during sleep. Others believe dreams are symbolic stories or metaphors we tell ourselves that represent personal and social mythology. Others believe that dreaming is one of the ways that people reflect on and make sense out of their waking life.

What Is Dreamwork?

Virtually every culture has believed dreams carry important messages. To the ancient Greeks, dreams were great healers. People who were sick slept in special healing temples in hopes of receiving therapeutic dreams from the gods. The *Talmud*, the Hebrew sacred book of practical wisdom, states clearly that the Jews gave great importance both to the dream and to the dream interpreter. Mohammed began writing the *Koran* after an angel visited him in a dream.

Tibetan Buddhists see no distinction between dreaming and waking and consider all of life a dream.

Plato saw dreams as a release for fervent inner forces. Hippocrates thought dreams were windows on illness and that normal dream content indicated a state of wellness and bizarre content a state of illness. Aristotle believed that the beginning of illness could be felt in dreams before actual symptoms appeared. Likewise, Artemidorus of Daldi, a physician in the Middle Ages, believed that dreams were like magnifying glasses that detected the small beginnings of physical illness.

Artemidorus wrote the first Western dream book in the second century, and the dreams recorded were remarkably similar to contemporary ones. Ghengis Khan is reported to have received his battle plans from his dreams, while Hannibal attributed the battle plan to attack Rome over the Alps with elephants as something that came to him in a dream.

During the late Middle Ages, dreams began to fall into disfavor among Christians in spite of the fact that throughout the Bible, God spoke directly to people through dreams and visions. St. Francis of Assisi founded the Franciscan Order as a dream directive from Christ.

In the United States, the traditional Iroquois were (and are) a people of dreams. Children were taught that dreams were the most important source of practical and spiritual guidance. The people of an Iroquois village began each day with dream sharing. The entire village became involved in dreamwork, especially if a dream seemed to contain a warning of death or disease. "Big" dreams were thought to come about in one of two ways. During sleep, the dreamer would have an out-of-body experience and travel to many places, past, present, and future. Alternatively, the dreamer could receive a visit from a spiritual being. Dreams were considered to be central to healing by providing insight into the causes of illness, often before physical symptoms appeared. Dreams continue to be important tools for many traditional healers in the Native American population.

Among indigenous peoples, shamans are recognized as dream counselors but not as "experts" in the Western sense. They are often called to their vocation by dreams.

Shamans have a special relationship with the dreamworld, and through dreams are able to look into the future, communicate with spirits, and clarify the meaning of other's dreams.

In 1900, Sigmund Freud wrote *The Interpretation of Dreams* and proposed that dreaming might represent a unique avenue by which unconscious motivation could be explored. Freud's theory was that dreams were disguised wish fulfillments of infantile sexual needs, which were repressed by censors in the waking mind. Freud's protege, Carl Jung, believed that humans were spiritual rather than instinctual and saw dreams as a compensatory mechanism with the function of restoring psychological balance. Jung said that the conscious and unconscious minds speak entirely different languages. The conscious mind is analytical, critical, and rational while the unconscious mind thinks metaphorically, in similes, symbols, and intuitively.

In a society that discounted dreams, Sigmund Freud introduced the concept of therapeutic dreamwork. He and his followers, however, began to associate dreams with illness rather than wellness, and reserved dream interpretation for professionals, who were deemed the only people competent to understand the latent content of dreams. This approach said, in effect, that individuals were not the experts on their own dreams. In contrast, Carl Jung stated that he "avoided all theoretical points of view and simply helped the patients to understand the dream-images by themselves, without application of rules and theories. .... That is how dreams are intended." Many contemporary therapists believe that dreams belong to individuals and they are the final authority on the meaning of their own dreams. This viewpoint is not to minimize the fact that the meaning of many dreams is obscure and that other people may be able to help unlock hidden meaning.

Dr. Nathaniel Kleitman is considered to be the father of modern scientific dream research. In 1957, he and Eugene Aserinsky identified rapid eye movement (REM), demonstrating the activity of the brain during sleep. This active sleep stage has consequently been called REM sleep. Today hundreds of sleep clinics operate in the United States, and sleep disorders constitute the second most common health complaint after the common cold.

How Does Dreaming Work?

At any point during sleep, our sleep can be characterized as either quiet or active changes in brain waves. Eye movements, muscle tone, and the presence of dreams are used to define the two states. The quiet state is divided into three stages. Stage one is the transitional state between drowsy wakefulness and light sleep. Transitional sleep can be characterized as slow drifting eye movements and vivid, brief dream images. Stage two is genuine sleep and is characterized by unique patterns called "sleep spindles," which are waxing and waning brain waves. After 20–30 minutes, people sink into the third stage, delta sleep. Named after the regular, slow brain waves that are characteristic of this stage of quiet sleep, delta sleep lasts about 30–40 minutes, during which the muscles are relaxed, although most people make major postural adjustments every 5–20 minutes. Some dreaming occurs during delta sleep, but it is poorly recalled, not vivid or emotional, and generally pleasant. The sleep pattern then retraces the same stages in reverse order.

About 90 minutes after the onset of sleep, several abrupt physiological changes occur as the sleeper enters REM sleep, or the active state, for the first time of the night. It is the sleep phase of vivid, memorable dreaming. Brain waves become desynchronized in a fast activity pattern that is similar, but not identical, to that of the waking state. An accompanying profound loss of muscle tone throughout the body causes a general paralysis except for the muscles of the eyes, middle ear ossicles, and respiration. Sometimes people awaken partially from REM sleep before the paralysis fades away, so that their body is still paralyzed, though they are otherwise awake. Sleep paralysis, as this state is called, can occur as people are falling asleep (rarely) or waking up (more frequently). Although the sensation may be terrifying, especially at the first occurrence, sleep paralysis is harmless.

During REM sleep, breathing may accelerate to a panting pace, and the rhythm of the heart may speed up or slow down. Typically, men have erections and women experience vaginal lubrication during every REM cycle, regardless of dream content. It is not unusual for men to ejaculate and women to experience orgasm during this time. During REM sleep, the cells of our brains, which have fired steadily while we were awake, fire in a wild and erratic pattern. Some neuroscientists believe dreaming is the brain's attempt to impose meaning on these signals from random firings.

During a typical night's sleep, the average adult alternates between periods of REM sleep and quiet sleep at regular intervals four to six times each night. After the first REM period, the intervals between REM periods decrease throughout the night, while the length of each REM period increases. REM sleep is both the deepest and lightest stage of sleep. It is the stage when people are least likely to be aroused by environmental stimuli and it is also the stage when people are most likely to awaken spontaneously.

REM sleep is a primary means of brain development and maturation. Infants born 10 weeks prematurely spend 80 percent of the total sleep time in REM sleep and those born two to four weeks prematurely spend 60–65% in REM sleep. Full-term newborns spend about half of their sleeping time in REM sleep, which decreases to 30–35% by the age of two. REM sleep stabilizes at about 25% by 10 years of age and shows little change until people reach their 70s or 80s when it decreases to about

18%. Thus, the dreaming that occurs during REM sleep is thought to be an important source of internal stimulation necessary for proper maturation of the brain, much as physical exercise is important in the development of muscles. This theory, however, doesn't explain why dreaming continues after the brain has fully developed.

Deprivation of REM sleep does not lead to psychosis, bizarre behavior, or anxiety, as was once feared. The interference with REM sleep may come from alcohol, sedatives, caffeine, drugs, anxiety, or depression. The most important effect of REM deprivation is a dramatic shift in subsequent sleep patterns. Reduction of REM sleep for several nights is followed by earlier onset and longer and more frequent periods of REM sleep. The longer the deprivation of REM sleep, the larger and longer the REM rebound. This compensatory mechanism suggests that REM sleep is physiologically necessary.

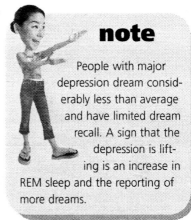

note

People with major depression dream considerably less than average and have limited dream recall. A sign that the depression is lifting is an increase in REM sleep and the reporting of more dreams.

Why Do We Dream?

Dreaming is a process of making broad connections. Dreams connect with recent experiences, old memories, and imagination. Dreaming makes connections not made during the waking state. The waking state tends to be guided by a specific task or goal, whereas dreaming tends to wander and form unique combinations. For example, people awake and thinking of a house may recall a specific house where they lived in the past. People dreaming and thinking of a house may see a generic house or a combination of several houses or even a hotel. During dreaming, consolidation of thoughts and memories occurs, and the bizarre twists and images of dreams often represent the processing and reclassifying of old information. Dream symbols bring together ordinary awareness and deeper levels of knowing. Since images mean different things to different people, it's the dreamer's dominant emotion that guides the dreaming process when choosing images in the memory related to that emotional concern. Dreams can be viewed as explanatory metaphors for the emotional state of the dreamer. "I leave my children in a house somewhere, and then I can't find them" may be a metaphorical description for the emotional state of guilt. If no single dominant emotion is present at the time, dreams may seem confused and almost random.

Jung believed that dreams are a remarkable way to reveal insights and solutions to deal with everyday problems encountered while awake. By and large, the language of dreams is anything but obvious, and for this reason it is easy to ignore the messages. What is bizarre to the conscious, rational mind is not so to the unconscious, which is rich in symbols. People who work on remembering and understanding their dreams often report that dreams provide insights for overcoming and resolving problems, and moving ahead.

While some dreams seem to be sequences of disconnected images, ideas, feelings, and sensations, others are story-like sequences that are dramatic and intricately detailed. They may have plots as coherent, funny, and profound as the best stories and plays. Some dreams are not told in a single episode and the dream series may conclude the following night, or some may run for as long as a TV soap opera.

Types of Dreams

Dreams offer nightly gauges on the dreamer's physical, emotional, and spiritual health. When disease begins to develop, dreams often provide warnings of specific problems before physical symptoms are apparent. The warning may be in the form of a broken heart, an exploding head, or limbs falling off. Such early diagnostic dreams are entirely natural and are reminders of how illness is related to one's entire being. Dreams give advice on preventive measures and ways to provide for one's well-being. Dreams frequently suggest specific courses of treatment for different problems. These suggestions may involve lifestyle changes, conventional medical treatments, alternative therapies, or counseling that address the hidden sources of disease. People may neglect the warnings but the unconscious is highly inventive in delivering the message in ways that make it harder and harder to ignore.

Nightmares are terrifying dreams with complex imagery and story lines that are usually vividly recalled. The most common scripts of nightmares include being chased by a monster, being naked in public, falling through space, losing something precious, and being unprepared for an important exam. Nightmares are especially terrifying because in dreams, anything is possible. Most typically, the dreamer is alone with no chance for escape.

Because REM sleep becomes more physiologically intense as sleep continues, most nightmares occur in the early morning hours. Some factors that seem to contribute to nightmare frequency are fever, stress, and troubled relationships. Traumatic events can trigger a long-lasting series of recurrent nightmares. Alcohol, drugs, and some medications that suppress REM sleep can cause an increase in nightmares. The person sleeps soundly for the first five or six hours with little dreaming. When the effect of the substance has worn off, the brain makes up for the lost REM time. As a result, dreams are more intense than usual for the last few hours of sleep. L-dopa, used in the treatment of Parkinson's disease, and beta blockers, used in the treatment of cardiovascular disorders, seem to increase nightmares by increasing the activity during REM sleep.

Conscious dreaming, sometimes referred to as lucid dreaming, is being aware that one is dreaming during the experience. People in this unusual state of consciousness are simultaneously aware of their bodies lying on a bed, aware of the content of their dreams, and aware of watching themselves dreaming. Conscious dreaming may be triggered by various things such as doing something impossible in the dream like flying or walking on water. Likewise, auditory signals such as a doorbell or a siren may startle people into becoming aware they are dreaming. Individuals who wish to explore and use dreams constructively in their lives can learn techniques to increase their conscious dreaming time.

Precognition is the condition of knowing about an event before it actually occurs. Precognitive dreaming involves seeing people and situations from the future and is an event where individuals are not bound by space-time. As people learn to recall their dreams and record them in a dream journal, they often begin to recognize and work with precognitive material in their dreams. Precognitive dreams may indicate what may happen if certain courses of action are pursued or they may show a precise event that cannot be altered.

Making Meaning, and Healing, for Our Dreams

Until recently, Western societies have discouraged dreamwork and dream sharing. When dreams are recalled, the significance is often minimized. People tend to remember only bits and pieces from dreams and often jumble together parts from several dreams into a single confused story. By the time individuals are fully awake they have forgotten 90%, if not more, of their nighttime adventures. Thus, the remembered dream is often different from the fuller dream experience.

By paying closer attention to dreams, people often gain greater access to their inner lives. Some of the world's most successful business executives never make a decision until they have had a chance to let it pass through their minds during sleep, allowing solutions to come during dreams. The first step in making sense of a dream is to own it. It belongs solely to the dreamer and is a personal story. Although many books have been written about dream symbols, they are best understood by the dreamer. Dreaming about a horse may be a symbol of comfort and security because the person always had a horse when she was growing up. A horse for another person may be a symbol of terror because he was kicked by a horse as a young child. A horse for another person may be a symbol for a challenge since she has wanted to learn to ride for some time. Thus, dream dictionaries do not have the answers to people's dream symbols; they are personal images taken from one's life representing one's unique experiences.

Dreams can be immensely useful in gaining self-knowledge. Psychologist Ernest Rossi has proposed that an important function of dreaming is integration of split-off parts of one's personality. According to Rossi:

> In dreams we witness something more than mere wishes; we experience dramas reflecting our psychological state and the process of change taking place in it. Dreams are a laboratory for experimenting with changes in our psychic life. ... This constructive or synthetic approach to dreams can be clearly stated: Dreaming is an endogenous process of psychological growth, change, and transformation.

The Tibetan Buddhist Tarthang Tulku writes:

> Experiences we gain from practices we do during our dream time can then be brought into our daytime experience. For example, we can learn to change the frightening images we see in our dreams into peaceful forms. Using the same process, we can transmute the negative emotions we feel during the daytime into increased awareness. Thus we can use our dream experiences to develop a more flexible life.

Tools for Dream Control

Journaling helps to mobilize intuition as people begin to understand their personal symbols. Because the dream journal is intensely personal, it should be kept private unless the dreamer chooses to share it with others. The entries should be dated so they can be correlated to significant life events in the present or future and recurring themes, places, and situations should be noted.

Giving dreams titles or headlines like a newspaper headline often reveals a dream message that may be otherwise overlooked. People are encouraged to go back over their journals at regular intervals to note connections between dreams and waking events.

In the midst of nightmares, people who realize they are dreaming frequently choose to wake up. Many therapists believe, however, that the essential issue is to discover what elements from the past, mixed with current events are creating the nightmare. Insight into the source of the nightmare can help people face and overcome the terror while remaining in the dream. Nightmares can be transformed into more pleasant experiences. People are encouraged to remember that nothing in their dreams can hurt them.

Conscious dreaming, as a form of mental imagery, has potential to aid in the promotion of health and in the healing process. Evidence supports the idea that the vividness of mental imagery determines how strongly it affects physiology. Dreams are the most vivid form of mental imagery most people experience, and therefore, they are also likely to be a source of highly effective healing imagery.

Reframing Nightmares

You need not seek professional help for bad dreams unless they frequently disrupt your sleep. Other distress signals include regular bouts of fatigue or depression when you wake up or consistently feeling worse than when you went to bed. Remember, nothing in your dreams can hurt you. During a nightmare, reframing the situation you are dreaming, to try to resolve whatever unconscious material is causing the nightmare. Some suggestions are given below. Alternatively, nightmares can be managed through a process called dream reentry, which is practiced in the waking state. Begin by selecting the nightmare to relive, and then come up with alternative ways of acting in the nightmare to transform the events into a more enjoyable experience. Relive the nightmare in imagination, incorporating the new action, and continue on with the dream until you see the result of your new behavior.

Being Chased

Response: Stop running and face the chaser, which may cause it to disappear. If not, try to talk and reconcile with the person or animal. Alternatively, ask the adversary what you are running away from.

Being Attacked

Response: Demonstrate your readiness to defend yourself, rather than giving in or running away. Then try to talk with the attacker in a soothing manner. Alternatively, enlist friendly and cooperative dream characters to help overcome the threatening character.

Falling

Response: Rather than waking up, go with it, relax, and land gently. Think about landing in a pleasant and interesting place. Alternatively, transform falling into flying.

Trapped or Paralyzed

Response: Relax and tell yourself you are dreaming. Go along with images or things that happen to the body, because none of it can be harmful in reality. Adopt an attitude of interest and curiosity about what happens.

Being Unprepared for an Exam or Speech

Response: Leave the exam room or the lecture hall. Alternatively, answer the text questions creatively or give a spontaneous talk on any topic of interest. The key is in transforming the experience into one that is fun.

Being Naked in Public

Response: Remember, modesty is a public convention and dreams are private experiences. Have fun with the idea. Try having everyone else in the dream remove their clothing also.

IMPROVING DREAM RECALL

■ Clearly declare to yourself the intention to remember your dreams when you lie down to sleep.

■ Have your tools, notebook and pen or tape recorder, at your bedside.

■ If you awaken during the night while dreaming, record your dream immediately. Use a penlight to see if you do not wish to disturb your partner. If you tell yourself that you can go back to sleep and catch the dreams later, you will probably find you are wrong.

■ When you awaken in the morning, at first lie quietly before jumping out of bed. Then write whatever you remember, even if only one word or scene.

■ If you wake with no dream memories, move your body back into the position you were in as you began to awaken and you will be more likely to recall your most recent dream.

■ Don't censor your dreaming and don't try to interpret right away. Bizarre, weird, or trivial dreams may become important later.

■ Pay attention to your feelings. They are often your best guide to the dream's meaning and urgency.

■ Keep a journal for a month of the dreams you do remember. Look for important ideas or themes running through the dreams.

■ The more you practice these skills, the more dreams you will remember.

Cultivating Healing Dreams

Dreams are the doorway into the unconscious, which is also a domain of healing. Just as guided imagery can be used to direct people's attention to specific areas or organs of the body, dreams too can become a healing tool.

■ One half hour before bedtime, find a quiet place.

■ Pay attention to the sounds and sensations of the outside environment as nature begins to settle down to rest.

- Spend a few minutes journaling the experiences and feelings you had during the day.

- Review your accomplishments of the day.

- Dwell for a moment on loving yourself and others with whom you interacted today.

- If you had conflict with others, put those thoughts and feelings away for now.

- Imagine yourself as part of the universe and feel a connection with all living things.

- Allow one issue of present concern to surface to your conscious mind.

- Ask for answers, solutions, or healing as you sleep and dream.

- On awakening, remember your previous night's request and let the answers come to your conscious mind.

Dream Incubation

A similar process is called dream incubation, which is a somewhat more deliberate format. Examples of the type of requests to make of our dreams are: How can I heal myself? Which path shall I choose? How can I solve (state problem)? How can I improve my relationship with (name)? How can I make (state project) a success? Should I do (state proposed action)? What shall I do now?

TRY IT YOURSELF: CULTIVATING A DREAM

1. Choose an important matter that you wish to explore.

2. Write down a short, simple question about which you want to know.

3. Meditate on the question for a few minutes. Repeat the question several times, followed by, "I give thanks for the answer, which will be in a dream that I remember."

4. Envision yourself awakening, remembering, and receiving an answer.

5. Write the question again.

6. Place the paper with the question on it beneath your pillow.

7. Upon awakening, follow the process in the TRY THIS box on improving dream recall.

8. Watch for extra information that may come later during the day.

9. Do not give up if you don't succeed immediately.

Dream Sharing

Sharing dreams with another person or with a group can provide a variety of insights into the many levels of the dream. Dream sharing also builds a sense of community as people discover they have a great deal in common. If you are sensitive and empathic and you have good listening, communication, and group skills, you can facilitate a dream-sharing group.

If you want each member of the group to have time to work on a dream at every session, you will have to limit your numbers to six or eight. Members should be asked to make a commitment to attend regular sessions over a set time, usually for no less than six weeks. A typical group session is two to three hours. Dream sharing requires mutual trust and respect. If people are going to share their innermost thoughts, they must have the assurance that they are in a place where they are protected and supported. The dream is always honored as a topic worthy of attention and thought. The protocol of dream sharing is as follows:

- All members are given an opportunity to share dreams if they choose, but are never pressured to do so.
- Dreams shared within the group should not be told to outsiders without the dreamer's permission.
- Sharing dreams does not mean giving up the right to privacy. Dreamers are free to share as much or as little about their dream or personal life as they wish.
- You are the final authority on the meaning of your dream.
- You cannot tell anyone else what her or his dream is about. You can only tell them what it would mean to you if it were your dream.

Even without a full understanding of what dreams signify, we can use their stories to know ourselves better. For many people—and you can be one of them—dreams really do come true.

The Absolute Minimum

- Dreaming is both physiologically and psychologically necessary; from its earliest points, history records mankind's fascination with dreaming, and theories of their significance vary as widely as dreams themselves.

- You can control your dreams: with a conscious will some practice, and perhaps collaboration with others, you can turn aside nightmares and seek psychological revelation and healing.

Resources

- Association for the Study of Dreams

    www.asdreams.org

- The Lucidity Institute

    www.lucidity.com

- Dream Gate

    www.dreamgate.com

- Sleep Home Pages from Brain Information Service

    bisleep.medsch.ucla.edu

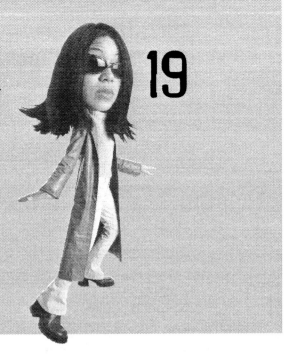

19

Biofeedback

Biofeedback is a method for learned control of physiological responses of the body. It is a relaxation technique using electronic equipment to amplify the electrochemical energy produced by body responses. Through conscious awareness, biofeedback provides perceptible information that you can use to gain voluntary control over various physiological processes.

What Is Biofeedback?

The experimental data to support the feasibility of learned control of our physiology through biofeedback first appeared in the 1950s. In 1961, experimental psychologist Neal Miller proposed that the involuntary nervous system was trainable, contrary to beliefs about human physiology at the time. As psychologists and physiologists continued this research, it became clear that dramatic gains could be achieved by using biofeedback information to assist people suffering from specific conditions, including headaches, ulcers, hypertension, and many other stress-related illnesses. The result of this work was the creation of biofeedback therapy, now widely used by both conventional and alternative practitioners. With the advent of computers, the technology has become even more powerful.

Biofeedback does not belong to any particular field of heath care but is used in many disciplines including nursing, psychology, social work, chiropractic, medicine, dentistry, physical therapy, rehabilitation, psychiatry, respiratory therapy, occupational therapy, physician assistant, exercise physiology, and sports medicine. Since 1980, all biofeedback therapists must have certification from the Biofeedback Certification Institute of America (BCIA). Licensed RNs are accepted with an AA degree, while all other applicants must hold a bachelor's degree or higher in one of the approved health care fields. Certification requires 60 hours in instructional biofeedback education as well as 140 hours in clinical experience. When applicants meet the requirements, they are allowed to sit for a qualifying examination that consists of both written and practical assessment. The BCIA provides directories of certified practitioners throughout the United States.

How Does Biofeedback Work?

The nervous system has two major components—voluntary and involuntary or autonomic. The voluntary component is totally under a person's control. If someone decides to stand, the brain sends a message to the appropriate muscle groups, and the person stands. In contrast, the autonomic nervous system functions without conscious thought. Although people may be able to change their rate of respiration, for example, they are not able to stop breathing indefinitely.

People receive biofeedback from their bodies all the time. When they do not eat, they feel hungry. When they run, they get winded. When they experience stress, their muscles tense. Other types of biofeedback are more difficult to discern. With the use of technology, however, people can learn to adjust their thought processes to control bodily processes such as blood pressure, temperature, muscle tension, bronchial dilation, gastrointestinal functioning, and brain wave activity. The concept is simple: If individuals can develop sensory awareness of an involuntary function, they can learn to sense it. For example, if skin temperature in the hands is converted into an audible signal, the beeps give one's ears and brain feedback. As people learn to dilate the arteries in their hands, thus raising skin temperature, the beeps speed up, providing instant feedback on what is occurring in the body. Biofeedback teaches people what it feels like to be relaxed internally so they can re-create the feeling whenever they choose.

The Tools of Biofeedback

Biofeedback instruments are highly sensitive electronic devices that monitor physiological processes. Signals from the body are amplified by the instrument and converted into usable information. The instruments may have meters, tones, or a computer display that presents the information to the patient. Temperature or thermal feedback is a primary tool for general relaxation training and treatment of specific vascular diseases. Blood flow in the hands responds to stress and relaxation, and the client learns to relax by watching the rise and fall of finger temperature. Electrodermal response (EDR) or galvanic skin response (GSR) feedback devices measure sweat gland activity of the fingertips or palm. This response is highly sensitive to emotions and thoughts.

It is used in general relaxation training, helping people reduce the impact of significant stressors, and in treating excessive sweating. Electromyography (EMG) feedback measures muscle tension with sensors placed on the skin over appropriate muscles. EMG feedback is used for general relaxation training and is the primary tool for the treatment of tension headache, pain reduction, and muscle spasm or paralysis due to injury or stroke. Sensors on the fingers provide pulse feedback, which is used for people experiencing anxiety, hypertension, and some cardiac arrhythmias. Respiratory resistance biofeedback measures the rate, volume, and rhythm of respiration and is useful in both asthma and the hyperventilation of anxiety and panic attacks. Electroencephalograph (EEG) records information about brainwave activity from sensors placed on the scalp. Changes in brain waves reflect changes in attention as well as in states of arousal from sleep to alert wakefulness. This type of feedback is used for mind quieting, attention control, insomnia, pain control, and substance abuse treatment. Cardiovascular (EKG) feedback is available through portable heart-rate monitors to augment a person's ability to control heart rate. In addition to being used by persons with cardiac disease, many professional athletes use this system to aid in their training. Sensors can now measure and report the activity of the internal and external rectal sphincters for the treatment of fecal incontinence, the activity of the detrusor muscle of the urinary bladder for the treatment of urinary incontinence, as well as esophageal motility and stomach acidity.

The Process of Biofeedback

After the desired mode of treatment is determined for the specific disorder, electrodes are attached to the person in the area to be monitored. These electrodes feed the information to a computer that registers the results either with a sound tone that varies in pitch or speed or on a visual monitor. EEG measurements produce a kind of video game of brainwaves. The human brain produces different brain waves during various states of consciousness. Beta waves are associated with normal or waking consciousness; alpha waves are produced in an altered or relaxed state of consciousness; and theta and delta waves are associated with unconscious and sleeping states. When the patient produces waves associated with concentration, the game speeds up. The game slows down when brainwaves associated with daydreaming are produced. This type of computer system can make learning control of body processes more interactive and fun, especially for children.

A biofeedback therapist leads the patient in mental exercises to help the person reach the desired result such as muscle relaxation or contraction or more of the alpha brain waves. Through trial and error, trainees eventually learn how to control the inner mechanism involved. Training typically requires 8–10 sessions, although people with long-term or severe disorders may require more sessions. Patients are expected to practice the skill 15–20 minutes a day throughout the training period to incorporate into their daily lives what they have learned.

Like other forms of therapy, biofeedback is more useful for some clinical problems than for others. Biofeedback is the preferred treatment in Raynaud's syndrome and in certain types of fecal and urinary incontinence. It is one of several preferred treatments for tension headaches, migraine headaches, irritable bowel syndrome, muscle reeducation, bruxism, temporomandibular joint syndrome (TMJ), and attention deficit disorder. Biofeedback is effective intervention in asthma, substance abuse, anxiety, cardiac arrhythmias, essential hypertension, epilepsy, and chronic pain syndromes.

TRY IT YOURSELF: MIND CONTROL OF MUSCULAR STRENGTH

1. Face your partner. Put your right hand on your partner's shoulder, palm up.

2. Clench your fist, and hold your arm straight.

3. Have your partner grasp your elbow with both hands and pull down while you resist. The pull needs to be gradual until you both get a sense of how much force is needed to bend your arm.

4. Now imagine you are a fire engine or pump. You are rooted to the earth and are drawing water up and it is pushing through your arm and out of your fingers at high speed with tremendous force—with such force that nothing can bend your arm.

5. Then place your arm again on your partner's shoulder, this time with the fingers outstretched, holding onto the feeling and the image of the pump pushing water through your arm with great force.

6. Ask your partner once more to apply gradual force to bend your arm. You will need to apply a little muscle power, but will find you can relax and hold steady with much less effort than before.

How Do I Start Using Biofeedback?

Certified biofeedback therapists, many of whom are nurses, help interpret signals from monitoring devices while leading their patients through physical and mental exercises to achieve the desired change in the body function being measured. Biofeedback creates a greater awareness of specific body parts and their functions. With training, you can regulate these functions. Biofeedback helps people to relieve or eliminate symptoms, provides an internal locus of control, and helps them reduce their own health care costs.

THE ABSOLUTE MINIMUM

■ Through learned control of the autonomic nervous system, biofeedback offers a way to control symptoms of chronic illnesses and everyday stress.

RESOURCES

- Association for Applied Psychophysiology and Biofeedback, Biofeedback Certification Institute

  www.aapb.org

- Association for Integrative Medicine

  www.integrativemedicine.org

- Society for the Study of Neuronal Regulation

  www.ssnr.com

20

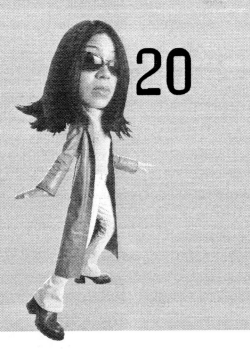

Movement-Oriented Therapies

A number of therapies focus on movement, body awareness, and breathing, and their purpose is to maintain health as well as to correct specific problems. This chapter presents two Eastern movement-oriented therapies: Qigong and T'ai Chi; and three Western movement-oriented therapies: the Alexander Technique, the Feldenkrais Method, and the Trager Approach. A major principle of these therapies is that awareness has to be experienced rather than taught, which then may lead to a more effective use of one's whole self.

The goal of all movement therapies is the retraining of one's body to improve coordination and balance, to release and change postural faults, and to relieve structural and functional stress.

How Do Movement-Oriented Therapies Work?

Like most alternative treatment, movement-oriented therapies aim to control and improve the flow of energy through the body. The "forms," or sequences of movements, are specifically designed to stimulate pressure points all along the body, and to encourage deep, rhythmic breathing, which fills the body with life-giving qi. The ultimate goal is to strengthen the flow of qi through the body to promote health and well-being. When qi is flowing in balance, the body stays healthy, resistant to disease, and can activate its own healing efforts.

The human body is viewed as a remarkable instrument, capable of responding with flexibility and resilience. But as the years pass, people often develop habitual reactions, beliefs, and movement patterns that cause physical and mental strain. Typically these habits manifest themselves by tight muscles, collapsed posture, or a lack of mobility. When muscles are working overtime, people eventually feel tight, tense, heavy, or tired. The sources of these problems are many—injury, illness, or stress. Lifelong misuse of muscles arises from sitting, standing, or walking incorrectly, or too much sitting and too little walking. For example, after years of walking incorrectly, back or knee problems can occur. A knee replacement is a temporary solution only, because the real problem lies not in the knee, but in the way the person moves from the hip. Movement-oriented practitioners believe the only lasting remedy is in reeducating the body to walk correctly to avoid injuring the knee. Likewise, back problems can be eliminated by learning appropriate ways of moving.

Sensory-movement activities are used to increase a person's sense of postural awareness, free from habitual patterns, and restoration of the proper use of muscles. Practitioners lead students though movements to enable them to discover a more fluid range of motion. As people develop new, alternative ways of moving, they experience positive sensory feelings and learn what it is like to be freer and lighter. The goal is to teach people how to move with minimum effort and maximum efficiency through increased consciousness of how their bodies work.

Almost anyone can participate in movement-oriented therapies. Movement therapies can be learned by the young and old, by the physically challenged or physically fit, and by those in good health, and those recovering from long-term injury or illness. In China, 80-, 90-, and 100-year-old people get up every morning before dawn and go out to the parks to practice Qigong or T'ai Chi, even in the middle of winter. These Eastern practices can be done alone, in pairs, or in large groups.

Qigong

Qigong, also spelled as Chi Kung, Chi Gong, or Chi Gung, is pronounced "chee goong." Qigong is a Chinese discipline, consisting of breathing and mental exercises that may be combined with modest arm movements. *Qi* is the term for vital energy and life force and *gong* means work or discipline. Qigong can be translated as "mastery of qi," "cultivation of energy," "air energy," "breath work," and "energy work." People discover how to generate more energy and conserve what they have in order to maintain health or treat illness.

Written records on Qigong go back 4,000 years. For almost all of that time, this practice remained a closely guarded family secret, available only to the elite classes in China. This discipline was handed down covertly and was not revealed until the beginning of the 20th century. In the late 1970s, the Chinese government funded several scientific studies of Qigong, which had been banned during the Cultural Revolution as superstitious practice. When a scientific basis was established, the government added Qigong to the list of treatment methods offered in Traditional Chinese Medicine hospitals.

Qigong is an easy and nontiring exercise that contains sets of moves designed to gather qi. Most people spend 30 minutes a day doing the exercises and another 30 minutes in meditation. Some forms are quite complex. For example, Wild Goose Qigong has two sections with 64 movements in each section. While it is difficult to learn, Wild Goose Qigong is exceptionally beautiful. In China, the goose is considered to be a marvelous creature that flies high into the clouds to gather cosmic energy and information and bring it to earth. Guo Lin Gong is a walking form of Qigong that is practiced in China particularly by people with cancer. Improvements have been documented in a wide range of conditions such as stroke, hypertension, spinal cord injuries, multiple sclerosis, joint disease, cerebral palsy, headaches, and many forms of cancer.

T'ai Chi

T'ai Chi, sometimes spelled as taiji, is pronounced "teye chee." T'ai Chi is a discipline that arose out of Qigong, and combines physical fitness, meditation, and self-defense. Literally translated, it means "great ultimate fist" and is sometimes translated as "supreme boxing" or "root of all motion." Although it is considered a martial art, T'ai Chi is mainly practiced today as a health discipline.

T'ai Chi, a modern offshoot of Qigong, was created by a Taoist priest in the 14th century. T'ai Chi gained popularity in the United States in the 1960s as people explored alternatives to conventional medicine. Some experts estimate that more than 800 million people practice Qigong or T'ai Chi internationally—nearly 20 percent of the world's population.

Qigong and T'ai Chi consist of soft, slow, continuous movements that are circular in nature. When practiced by a master, the movements are so slow and fluid that they look like swimming in air. The softness of movements develops energy without nervousness. The slowness of movements requires attentive control that quiets the mind and develops one's powers of awareness and concentration. The continuous circular nature of the movements develops strength and endurance. Yin and yang refer to the balance of forces in the universe. T'ai Chi movements are designed to express these forces in balanced form by pairs of opposites. For example, a motion that ultimately involves turning to the right often begins with a small movement to the left. In Qigong, students learn to sense their qi and follow it as it moves around the body. As they become more skillful, they learn to strengthen their qi and direct it to specific areas of the body that are weak or ailing.

For most people, Qigong and T'ai Chi are personal disciplines. Most practitioners spend 30–60 minutes a day doing the exercises. With more intensive practice over many years, some become masters. A T'ai Chi master is generally one who has exceptional skill in doing the form or in using the principles in boxing and in life. A Qigong master is one who has developed the ability to emit healing energy and has achieved proven success in healing with qi. Masters may also have qualities that are generally considered supernatural in the areas of special insight and spiritual transcendence. Rarely, if ever, will a true master call herself or himself a master. Rather, they say that "the practice is the teacher" and that "the qi is the teacher."

It is difficult to learn Qigong or T'ai Chi from a book, audiotape, or video. While simple forms may be grasped this way, the more complex forms are nearly impossible to learn without a teacher's guidance. In the Chinese tradition, one chooses and remains devoted to a teacher. The teacher-disciple relationship is revered as the only path to advanced skill. The honor and reverence that is bestowed on the teacher is part of the belief system that empowers the disciple.

Yang is the most popular form of T'ai Chi and was developed in the early 20th century by Yang Cheng Fu. It is composed of 108 separate motions, which can take 6–12 months to learn. When they are strung together, the result is a cross between slow-motion shadow boxing and dancing. Each movement has a name, like "repulse the monkey," "the snake creeps down," "the white crane spreads its wings," or "parting the wild horse's mane," which describes what it looks like or what purpose it serves. For example, when one is trying to concentrate, monkey thoughts are distractions. As the monkey is pushed away, the person is not allowing distractions to take attention away from the process of the moment. T'ai Chi also has breathing exercises for the purpose of improving and strengthening the flow of qi. One form involves reversed breathing, which is contracting the stomach with the in-breath and expanding the stomach with the out-breath. The benefits of T'ai Chi are seen in conditions such as hypertension, osteoporosis, and arthritis. T'ai Chi can decrease stress and fatigue, improve mood, and increase energy. It is especially helpful in improving balance in older adults, which decreases the risk of falls.

The Alexander Technique

The Alexander Technique is a method to improve posture and movement dysfunctions that can lead to pain and disease. It is designed to reduce and eliminate body misuse in daily activities especially in respect to the head, neck, and shoulders.

The Alexander Technique was developed more than a century ago by F. M. Alexander, an Australian actor who had lost his voice while performing. He carefully watched himself while speaking and observed that undue muscular tension accounted for his vocal problem. He sought a way to eliminate that restriction, and the technique he developed focused on correcting the misuse of the neuromuscular activity of the head, neck, and spine. The Alexander Technique is taught in the curriculum of music conservatories, theater schools, and universities throughout the world, as a foundation for improved health and creative exploration. It is also a useful tool to help people, able-bodied and disabled, maximize their movement potential.

The North American Society of Teachers of the Alexander Technique (NASTAT) is the certifying body for practitioners. A NASTAT-certified teacher must complete a 1,600-hour training program over a minimum of three years. The emphasis of the training is on observation and modification of human movement patterns to identify and eliminate sources of movement dysfunction.

The Alexander Technique includes simple movements that improve balance, posture, and coordination and relieve pain. During a session, the client goes through a series of standing and seated exercises while the practitioner applies light pressure to points of contraction in the body. The techniques help people learn how to use their bodies with less tension and more awareness. The recommended course is 30 lessons, depending on the client's participation and initial level of functioning.

The Feldenkrais Method

The Feldenkrais Method uses gentle movement and directed attention to improve movement and enhance functioning. The physics of body movement are combined with an awareness of the way people learn to move, behave, and interact.

The Feldenkrais Method was developed by Moshe Feldenkrais (1904–1984), a Russian-born Israeli physicist, mechanical engineer, and judo expert. After suffering crippling knee injuries, Feldenkrais used his own body as his laboratory and taught himself to walk again. In the process, he developed a system for accessing the power of the central nervous system to improve human functioning.

All Feldenkrais practitioners must complete 800–1000 hours of training over a period of three to four years. The main purpose of the training is for practitioners to develop a deep understanding of movement, to become aware of their own movement, to become skillful observers of movement in others, and to be able to teach other people to increase their awareness and improve their skills of movement.

The Feldenkrais Method consists of two parts—awareness through movement and functional integration. They are convenient labels for doing essentially the same thing in different ways. Awareness though movement is more like conventional exercises in format, with the teacher guiding a group class with words rather than by personal manipulation. The lessons consist of comfortable, easy movements that gradually increase in range and complexity designed for all levels of movement ability. Functional integration is a hands-on lesson that usually lasts 45 minutes to an hour and is performed with the client fully clothed and standing, sitting, or lying on a table. The practitioner touches and moves the client in gentle, noninvasive ways. The intent of this touch is to explore the person's responses to touch and movement, and then suggest alternative ways of moving.

Feldenkrais exercises are small, gentle movements, such as pelvic tilts—slowly and deliberately lifting the spine from the coccyx to the waist, one vertebra at a time. To be effective, the movements must be effortless. If exercise becomes painful, no learning takes place, because the brain is too focused on how to stop doing the painful activity. Feldenkrais exercises are said to improve flexibility, posture, range of motion, relaxation, ease of movement, physical performance, vitality, and well-being. They are also said to relieve joint pain, stress, muscle tension, low back pain, neck and shoulder pain, jaw pain, and headaches.

The Trager Approach

Developed in the early 1930s by Milton Trager, the Trager Approach was based on Trager's years of experience as a boxing trainer. He spent the next 50 years, first as a lay practitioner and later as a physician, expanding and refining his discovery. It is a method of movement reeducation designed to produce positive, pleasurable feelings and tissue changes by means of sensory-motor feedback loops between the mind and the muscles.

The Trager Institute provides training and certifies Trager practitioners. It takes an average of two years to complete the program's 269 hours of training and field work. Students learn the relationship between various groups of muscles and organs that produce patterns of posture and movement. The focus is on the mechanics of movement, the kinesthetic interaction, and principles of neuropatterning underlying movement.

The Trager Approach is a process of using motion in muscles and joints to produce particular sensory feelings. These feelings are relayed to the central nervous system and then, through the process of feedback loops, they trigger changes in the tissues. A Trager session takes 60–90 minutes with the client wearing a swimming suit and lying on a well-padded table. The practitioner touches in such a gentle rhythmic way that the person actually experiences the possibility of being able to move each part of the body freely and effortlessly. Because active participation of the client is discouraged, the passive body can freely learn new movements. Trager practitioners work in a meditative state they call "hook-up." This state allows the practitioner to connect deeply with the client in an unforced way, to remain continually aware of the slightest responses, and to work efficiently without fatigue.

Following this session, the student is given instruction in the use of mentastics, a system of simple, effortless movement sequences designed to maintain and even enhance the sense of lightness, freedom, and flexibility that was instilled during the treatment session. Mentastics, Dr. Trager's coined term for "mental gymnastics" is a powerful means of reinforcing positive changes. The Trager Approach is said to decrease various types of chronic pain, headaches, temporomandibular joint pain, improve muscle spasms, and aid in recovery from stroke and spinal cord injuries.

How Do I Begin Using Movement-Oriented Therapies?

Like most moderate physical activities practiced on a daily basis, T'ai Chi and Qigong can improve stability, agility, flexibility, stamina, and muscle tone. They are good exercise for people who are already in shape. But they can also be adapted for older adults, children, or people with injury or illness. The movements are gentle and put less stress on the body than do other exercises. The breathing exercises are a form of meditation that quiets the mind and reduces the negative effects of stress.

If you or others you know are healthy and wish to maintain your health, learning T'ai Chi or Qigong is highly recommended. Experienced practitioners spend at least 20 and up to 60 minutes in daily practice. To increase health, it is important to build up stamina over a period of time. If you are seriously ill, you may only be able to do the simple breath practices, as they focus on absorbing healing qi from the environment. When you can manage it, add simple hand gestures to the breathing. As you continue to improve, sit in a chair and do the hand motions, moving on to the standing and walking positions when you feel able.

Two common movements in T'ai Chi that are part of various sequences are the T'ai Chi fist and the T'ai Chi ball. Imagining a robin's egg in the center of each palm, the fist is formed by slowly curling one finger at a time around the egg, beginning with the little finger and ending with the thumb resting lightly on top. Throughout all the forms, frequent references are made to "picking up the ball." Visualize forming a ball out of the air and picking it up and moving with it. The ball is designed to help movements flow more easily.

Standing like a tree or the horse-riding stance contributes to a sense of rootedness and stability in the body. For this posture, position your legs wider than the shoulders and bend your knees, thus lowering your center of gravity closer to the earth. The top part of the body feels light while the lower half feels heavy. At first, the position may feel strenuous because the muscles in the legs have not been used in this way, but with practice, you will enjoy the feeling of stability it gives you. Next, bring your arms up as if embracing an invisible person, joining your fingertips in front of you. Slowly turn from side to side, letting your waist initiate the movement. Your legs should feel "soft," so that they follow the movement led by the waist. Your gaze should travel slowly across an imagined horizon.

T'ai Chi and Qigong are popular and available in most towns and cities. They are taught in health clubs, schools, YMCAs, community centers, hospitals, clinics, and other facilities. It is useful, in most cases, to begin with a teacher, so ask around to find a teacher whom others like, then observe a class or participate in a trial class. Some people try several teachers or forms before they find the one that meets their personal preferences.

As T'ai Chi and Qigong have become more popular, people can be found practicing in parks. In some cases, individuals prefer to have time alone in nature. Often, however, people are happy to have others join them, and frequently informal groups form. These groups may develop socially as people get to know one another and socialize after the practice.

The claims for the Alexander Technique, the Feldenkrais Method, and the Trager Approach focus more on enhancing well-being than on healing illness. They are designed to relieve muscle tension, increase relaxation, reduce stress, and alter poor habits of posture and movement in those who are healthy. Contact the appropriate associations (listed in the Resources section) to locate certified teachers of these techniques.

THE ABSOLUTE MINIMUM

■ Movement therapies offer Eastern and Western, ancient and modern approaches to the same goal: increased energy and stability of our bodies.

■ The benefits of movement therapies are most intensely experienced with working with a practitioner, who will help ensure that the movements are being performed correctly.

TRY IT YOURSELF: MOVING INTO YOUR CENTER

When starting T'ai Chi and Qigong, it is best to begin with simple exercises. Getting the body into alignment is an important part of these movement therapies. Stand with your feet shoulder-width apart, buttocks tucked in, spine straight, shoulder relaxed, knees unlocked, the head straight and resting lightly on top of the spine as if a string from the top of the head were gently suspending the body from above. Standing in this position, pay attention to your breathing, inhaling deeply and exhaling all the way out. Standing in this position, locate your tan t'ien (pronounced don tee-en). It is the body's center of gravity and stability, located about one-and-a-half inches below the navel and into the center of the body. T'ai Chi and Qigong teach people to find and maintain their center through movement, whereas in meditation and yoga, centering is found in stillness. The tan t'ien is considered to be the source of energy and, as you practice, you will find that all the movements begin to flow more easily if they begin from the tan t'ien.

FEEL YOUR QI

1. Stand with your feet shoulder-width apart, your knees slightly bent, your spine upright, and your shoulders relaxed. Breathe easily.

2. Start to flex or bounce gently at the knees.

3. Still bouncing, shift your weight back and forth from your right to left leg.

4. Keep your breathing relaxed and deep.

5. Begin to snap all of your fingers, flipping each one past your thumb.

6. Then, still bouncing and finger-snapping, twist at your waist, to the right, then to the left.

7. While you are doing all this, make your exhale a sigh of relief. Do five of these sighs in a slow, relaxed manner.

8. Now stop and close your eyes and turn your attention inward. Feel the buzzing, humming, or tingling sensation that is in your hands, legs, and body. This is qi. You are literally feeling the activity of the profound medicine you have produced within yourself.

RESOURCES

▓ East-West Academy of Healing Arts

www.eastwestqi.com

▓ Feldenkrais Guild of North America

www.feldenkrais.com

▓ North American Society of Teachers of the Alexander Technique (NASTAT)

www.Alexandertech.com

▓ The Trager Institute

www.trager.com

PART VI

SPIRITUAL THERAPIES

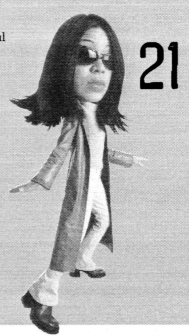

21

SHAMANISM

Shaman (pronounced SHAH-min) is a word from the Tungus people of Siberia. This term has been adopted widely by anthropologists to refer to those known in the West as "medicine men," "witch doctors," "witches," "magicians," and "seers." Not every kind of medicine person or witch doctor, however, is a shaman. A *shaman* is a woman or man who enters an altered state of consciousness, at will, to contact and utilize another type of reality to acquire knowledge and power to help other people. Shamans use ancient techniques to achieve and maintain well-being and healing for themselves and members of their communities, serving as a link between the worlds of matter and spirit. Shamanism is not a belief system. Rather, it is a broad umbrella covering ancient, indigenous, and holistic healing practices worldwide. For further information on Native American healers, see Chapter 5.

What Is Shamanism?

The origins of shamanism go back to Stone Age times, making it the oldest of all healing therapies. All over the world, evidence from ancient cave drawings and similar records support the conclusions that indigenous peoples shared a similar understanding of how the universe works, how to maintain health and strength, how to cope with serious illness, and how to deal with the trauma of death. One of the most remarkable aspects of shamanism is that concepts and treatment methods are similar in widely separated and remote parts of the planet among peoples isolated from one another. Anthropologists have studied shamanism in North, Central, and South America, Africa, Australia, Indonesia, Malaysia, Bali, Tibet, Korea, Siberia, and across Europe, and found that shamans functioned fundamentally in much the same way and with similar techniques worldwide. The basic uniformity suggests that, through trial and error, people arrived at the same conclusions.

Today, shamanism survives in less "developed" regions of the world in spite of the advent of Western scientific medicine. The field of holistic medicine is reclaiming many techniques long practiced in shamanism, such as visualization, altered state of consciousness, hypnotherapy, meditation, positive attitude, and stress reduction. Shamanic healing is rapidly gaining popularity among urban Americans as people turn back to the old cultures for help and guidance in finding a better balance with nature and with themselves. Shamanic practice and biomedical treatment are not in conflict. Contemporary shamans are perfectly willing to have their patients see a conventional physician, because the primary goal is wellness. Any kind of technological treatment or medication that will contribute to the strength of the patient is welcomed.

Becoming a Shaman

People discover in a wide variety of ways that their purpose in life is to become a shaman. Often potential healers have prophetic dreams about their future calling. The dream may even include details about locating a teacher and the length of the training. In some cases, people are led to shamanism through personal and private mystical experiences, while in other cases, they are drawn from the ranks of cured patients.

The journey from apprentice to shaman is illustrated in the following example of Native American shamans. The first step is "embracing personal history." This process includes working through old traumas, fears, anger, hate, abandonment, betrayals, and wounds. The purpose is to heal the emotions so that one is no longer controlled by them but rather, consciously guided by feelings. The second step is "facing death and making death an ally." This step means examining one's attitudes and beliefs to "put to death" any that are inaccurate or outdated. It includes remembering that bodies are temporary and will one day be claimed by death. It is moving beyond personal history and recognizing that all people are part of a family, village, tribe, city, country, and ultimately all humanity. The third step is "stopping the world," which involves clearing the mind of its mental garbage. The fourth step is "controlling the dream and finding new vision and purpose." This is the time to quest for vision and seek direct connection with the dream world and its spiritual teachers. The Vision Quest is part of many old world cultures and is a time when one fasts and prays in a sacred place, often a mountaintop, for up to four days and nights. The person prays for a vision and thus a reconnection with the Creator and Creation. Following the Vision Quest, the person is expected to make life changes that were called for. The fifth and final step is taking full responsibility for all of one's actions without guilt or shame. Apprentice shamans go through this path of transformation, as they become healers and helpers in service to other people.

Shamanic initiation is experiential and often gradual. Shamans must learn how to achieve the shamanic state of consciousness; they must become familiar with their own guardian spirits, and must successfully help others as a shaman. After learning the basic principles and methods, new shamans extend their knowledge and power by shamanic journeying. Many years of shamanic experience are necessary for the few shamans who become true masters of knowledge, power, and healing.

How Does Shamanism Work?

Shamanic healing is a manifestation of the personal power of the shaman, who uses altered states of consciousness, imagination, and environmental and spiritual guides to create an experience of healing within the patient.

Finding Harmony with the Environment

For the shaman, everything exists as part of an infinite web of life. Plants, stones, the earth herself, are all perceptive beings; they are all consciously aware and have a story to tell. In the shamanistic tradition, people communicate intimately and lovingly with "all their relations," as the Lakota would say, talking not just with other people, but also with animals, plants, and all the elements of the environment, including rocks and water. From the shaman's viewpoint, one's surroundings are not "environment," but family. A deep respect for all forms of life is present, with a great awareness of one's dependence on the environment. Shamans believe their powers are the powers of the animals, of the plants, of the sun, of the basic energies of the universe. They are expected to live in harmony with nature and to provide strength in daily life, and help save others from illness and death.

Drawing on Personal Power

In shamanism, the preservation of one's personal power is fundamental to well-being. Specific shamanic methods restore and maintain personal power and use it to help others who are weak, ill, or injured. In shamanism, the word medicine means vital force or energy. A person's medicine is their power, their knowledge, and their expression of their life energy.

Many shamans keep power objects, their medicine, in a medicine bundle. This bundle is normally kept wrapped up and is unrolled publicly only on ritual occasions. The objects inside are highly personal and, as with other matters of power, one does not boast of them because to do so might result in power loss. Almost any small object can be included, but the quartz crystal is highly prized among the shamans of North and South America, Australia, Southeast Asia, and elsewhere. Quartz crystals are six-sided stones that are usually transparent to milky white, and in a sense, appear to be "solidified light." The quartz crystal is considered the strongest power object and is viewed as a spirit helper. For thousands of years, shamans have used their quartz crystals for power in seeing and divination. Interestingly, in modern physics, the quartz crystal is also involved in the manipulation of power. Its remarkable electronic properties made it a basic component in early radio transmitters and receivers. Later, quartz crystals became basic components for modern electronic hardware such as computers and timepieces.

Controlling States of Consciousness

The Ordinary State of Consciousness (OSC) is an agreed-upon consensus of what reality is. This OSC, also called ordinary reality or simply "reality," is determined by every society and learned by individuals from childhood. Reality, then, is predetermined expectations. For example, in Western societies, people are not surprised when they put a card in a machine and money comes out. Another characteristic of Western ordinary reality is that it can be measured and quantified. Nonordinary realities are other levels of consciousness. They can be experienced during dreaming, or induced by drugs, fasting, sleep deprivation, or environmental factors. In Western society, this level of consciousness is often viewed as psychosis rather than another legitimate reality.

Shamans move, at will and with serious intention, between an Ordinary State of Consciousness and a Shamanic State of Consciousness (SSC). The SSC is an altered state of consciousness that may vary from a light to a deep trance. Shamans journey back and forth between these realities for the specific purpose of healing or in some manner aiding the community. Shamans operate in nonordinary reality or SSC only a small portion of the time, and then only as needed to perform shamanic tasks.

During this trance state, shamans' souls are believed to leave their bodies and ascend to either the upper world or lower world. Unlike the altered state of consciousness during dreaming, the SSC is a conscious waking state and at any time shamans can will themselves out of it, back into the OSC. The experience is like a waking dream in which shamans can control their actions and direct their adventures. Unlike a mind-altering drug experience, the SSC experience is not dependent on a chemically determined length of time, nor does it risk the possibility of being locked into a "bad trip."

Tapping the Imagination

Most indigenous people make little distinction between what Westerners call imagination and reality. Imagination is just as real and just as concrete as ordinary reality. In fact, most of the material things of the "real" world were someone's imagination first. Automobiles, televisions, and computers have come from the imaginary realm. In fact, logic and reason have always been preceded by imagination. Western people often ask whether the power animals and guardian spirits have is real or imagined. If the information that is received from power animals and guardian spirits empowers people, improves their lives, and helps them heal, the question does not apply. It is real because people's lives are changed.

The Shamanic Cosmology

Shamanic cultures throughout the world have a three-tiered cosmology or way of viewing the universe. The middle world is the world of OSC or ordinary reality. It is the world of matter and the world in which people live their daily lives. The lower world and the upper world are SSC worlds, nonordinary reality, or worlds of the spirit, not to be confused with heaven and hell. These worlds are just as real as the ordinary reality of the middle world.

The lower world is the world of power animals. These archetypical energies take the form of animal guides who have knowledge and wisdom to share and help people navigate through life. Power animals tend to provide practical help and guidance. The capability of power animals to speak to humans is taken as an indication of their power. The belief that shamans can shape-shift into the form of their power animal is common to many cultures. Sharing the identity of one's power animal varies among shamans. Some speak publicly about them while others fear that disclosing the animal's identity may cause it to leave the person. Many cultures believe that every person is born with a particular animal spirit that is to be their guide throughout life. A similar belief in Western cultures is that of guardian angels watching over people, especially children.

The upper world is the world of spirit guides. Spirit guides are beings that look more like people and are more familiar to most individuals. It is in the upper world that people meet their guardian angels. The help from spirit guides tends to be more general and philosophical in comparison to the practical help from the lower world. These worlds are complementary and equal, and neither is superior to the other.

Power animals and spirit guides teach people how to be empowered, improve their lives, and even heal themselves. One does not have to be a shaman to make contact with one's personal power animal and spirit guide. The most traditional method of accessing this nonordinary reality is the shamanic journey.

The Shamanic View of Health and Illness

The ability to maintain good health is a matter of power in the shamanic world view. If the body is power-filled, it resists the intrusion of external, harmful forces. No room is available for disease and illness in a power-filled body. Being power-full is like having a protective force field surrounding the body. Possession of guardian spirit power is also fundamental to health. From a shamanic point of view, illnesses usually are intrusions that break the force field of power-fullness. In some ways this concept is not too different from the biomedical concept of infection. Serious illness and other misfortunes are usually only possible when people are disspirited, meaning they have lost their power and their guardian spirits. This loss results in an inability to fight off unwanted intrusions. Illness is viewed as a separation from one's power, from one's guardians, from nature, from community, and from the Great Spirit. Even Western everyday language reflects this view when people say, "I'm having a low-energy day," or "I wasn't myself last night."

Severe trauma can result in soul loss, a natural survival mechanism. It is believed that a part of one's self or soul goes into hiding to ensure that the individual will survive the extreme stress. Western psychiatrists refer to this phenomenon as dissociation. Sometimes people's souls remain lost until they go through a process of soul retrieval. Symptoms of soul loss are an inability to focus and concentrate, a lack of connection to one's emotions, a feeling of being "spaced out" and not really present, a feeling of being an observer of life rather than a participant, or chronic depression. Soul retrieval brings buried memories and emotions back to the surface, much like the process of psychotherapy.

Healing as a Journey

Shamans may be called upon to help those who have become ill or those who have lost their power, their spirit guides, or even their souls. In such cases, shamans use the shamanic journey to recover what was lost. Shamans also journey to gather information to help and guide individuals or groups, solve problems, and answer questions. Shamans, by offering their total commitment to a patient for as long as several days, develop intense relationships that underscore the importance of caring as well as curing in the shamanic healing tradition. In old cultures, shamans would do the journeying for patients, but in today's world, anyone can experience a shamanic journey. It is through this process that people meet and talk with their power animals and spirit guides and restore their own power and self-healing.

Basic tools for entering the SSC prior to the shamanic journey are the drum, providing lower vibrations, and the rattle, providing higher vibrations. A drum beat at a steady 200 to 280 beats a minute serves as a focus for concentration and quiets the chattering mind. The pace of the drumbeat corresponds to theta brainwaves associated with the hypnotic state, facilitating the move into nonordinary reality. It is a remarkably safe practice for most people, because one can return to an ordinary state of consciousness at any time. Some people add dancing or chanting to the drum beat as another way to reach this altered state of consciousness.

Some shamans use teacher plants as a catalyst to the shamanic journey. Throughout the world are many teacher plants: peyote, San Pedro cactus, ayahuasca, psilocybin, and red and white mushrooms, for example. Shamans consider these plants to be gifts to be used with care and awareness. Their use is never intended to be recreational but rather as a part of a sacred ceremony.

Sometimes communities share in a group healing ceremony. An example is found among the indigenous people of Hawaii, who come together as a group and experience a forgiveness ritual before the shaman begins the healing work. Family and community members convey concern for the patient by their participation in the ritual. This process underscores the belief that no one lives in isolation but is connected to and affected by other people. When people join together in a show of community support, new levels of healing are possible.

TRY IT YOURSELF: YOUR OWN SHAMANIC JOURNEY

- Find a private, secure place where you will not be disturbed.

- Assume a comfortable position, either sitting or lying down. You may want to cover your eyes to block out room light.

- Set the intent of your journey—if you want to go to the upper or lower world with the intent to meet your guardian spirit or your power animal.

- Turn on a drumming tape. Let your body relax, and let it sink down into Mother Earth. Take a few deep, slow breaths. Let the drum beat become part of you; feel it resonate through your body.

- In your mind, bring yourself to a place in nature that is special for you, one that holds personal meaning. It might be a tree you climbed as a child, the lake you swam in on summer vacations, the place you now walk your dog. Imagine that place and go there in your mind. Feel the energy of that place.

- If you are going to the lower world, find a place you can enter the earth such as a hollowed out tree stump, an animal den, a cave, or whatever you want to imagine. When you enter the earth, you will be in a long cave. Take your time and follow it. Eventually it will open up into the lower world. Walk around and enjoy the beauty of the lower world. Explore. Soon you will come in contact with power animals. Introduce yourself. Dialogue with the animal, and ask what information the animal has for you.

- If you are going to the upper world, find a way to get up into the sky. You may climb a mountain or a tall beanstalk, use a hot air balloon, or even shape-shift into the form of an eagle and fly up. Eventually, you will come to the interface between the middle world and the upper world. Find a way through this interface, which is something like a membrane. The upper world is an ethereal, light, crystalline place. Explore. Soon you will meet your guardian spirit. Introduce yourself. Dialogue with the spirit, and ask what information the spirit has for you.

- Eventually, the journey has to end. It can end when you decide to end it, when no more information remains to be gained, or when the drum beat changes, signaling an end. Return home by the same path you took to get there.

- Allow the information to sink into your consciousness. It is best if you write the information down in a notebook, in a concrete form you will remember. The shamanic journey is much like a dream—it will leave you quickly. Writing it down is a method to keep the information you gained during the journey.

Finding Your Friendly Neighborhood Shaman

Albert Schweitzer reportedly once observed, "The witch doctor succeeds for the same reason all the rest of us [doctors] succeed. Each patient carries his own doctor inside him. They come to us not knowing this truth. We are at our best when we give the doctor who resides within each patient a chance to go to work." This belief is almost identical to Florence Nightingale's basic premise that healing is a function of nature that comes from within the individual.

A current example of a combination of the techniques of shamanism with biomedicine is the well-known work of Dr. O. Carl Simonton and Stephanie Matthews-Simonton in treating people with cancer. As part of their treatment, patients are taught to relax and visualize themselves on a walking journey until they meet an "inner guide," which is a person or animal. The patient then asks the guide for help in getting well. The process is similar to a shamanic journey and the meeting of a power animal.

Contemporary shamans work with today's Native American and other indigenous cultures. Their repertoire of curative powers now includes some modern and biomedical practices, and they may collaborate with conventional health care practitioners. Today, many shamans share their knowledge about healing with others, which has contributed to a recent renewal of interest in this oldest of healing therapies. Lectures, retreats, and weekend meetings, where shamans teach the principles of living in balance with nature, are now available to the general public.

Shamanism offers a chance for contemplation. Guides offer more in the way of introspection and insight than physical cure. A shamanic journey may increase your self-understanding, provide guidance for living, and foster a spiritual rejuvenation, all of which are important for the healing process.

Finding the Beat of Your Healing

In the old cultures, shamans would do the journeying while an apprentice or helper drummed. In today's world, it is more appropriate for each of us to learn to journey for ourselves and restore our own power. Personal power is believed to be basic to health and well-being. You may wish to meet in drumming circles every one or two weeks or you may prefer to work alone. Drumming tapes have been designed and produced for shamanic journeying. As in any other field of learning, it may be more effective to work firsthand with a professional during a workshop or retreat.

The shamanic journey begins with the drum. Among all the instruments used in healing, the drum produces some of the most powerful effects. Drumming has been used in organizations ranging from therapy groups and twelve-step programs to rehabilitation centers. Human bodies are multidimensional rhythm machines with everything pulsing in synchrony. Drumming can influence how strongly and harmoniously life moves within and around us.

In the shamanic tradition, healing is not just for the individual but also for the community. In shamanism, ultimately no distinction is made between helping others and helping yourself. By helping others, one becomes more powerful, self-fulfilled, and joyful. The broader purpose is the helping of humankind.

THE ABSOLUTE MINIMUM

- Shamans create healing and growth experiences in others through the use of their personal power, their ability to enter altered states of consciousness, and their harmony with the environment.

- By regarding healing as a journey and attempting to access your own shamanic qualities, you can create shamanic healing for yourself.

RESOURCES

- The Foundation for Shamanic Studies

  www.shamanism.org

- Eagle's Wing Centre for Contemporary Shamanism

  www.shamanism.co.uk

In This Chapter

- Exploring the ancient and modern links between religion, spirituality, and healing.

- Effective healing and lifestyle practices can be fostered by faith and religious observance.

- Ways to begin tapping the healing powers of faith.

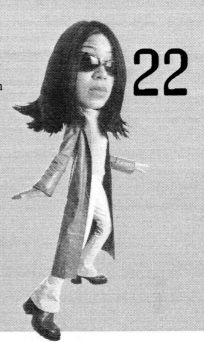

22

Faith and Prayer

Health care sciences have begun to demonstrate that faith and religious commitment may play a role in promoting health and reducing illness. Clinicians and researchers, as well as others, are becoming more interested in the connection between religious faith and survival. Increasingly, people are beginning to recognize that faith is good medicine.

Religion as a Healing Practice

Religion develops and changes over time and is composed of people's beliefs, attitudes, and patterns of behavior that relate to the supernatural—God, the Divine One, the Great Spirit, Creator, and so on. Religion usually includes a group of people who hold similar beliefs and participate in shared traditions. A community of religious people may or may not have a formal organizational structure.

The U.S. population would seem to be religious, with 95 percent of the general public expressing a belief in God and more than two-thirds claiming that they base their entire approach to life on their religious beliefs. For decades, surveys have found that more than 90% of Americans reportedly pray. Recently both *Time* and *Newsweek* devoted cover stories to the popular and sometimes controversial topic of prayer and religious healing. The *Newsweek* poll found that 54% of Americans pray daily, with 29% reporting that they pray more than once a day.

The History of Medicine and Religion

Until the last 200 years, medicine and religion were so thoroughly united that healers and priests were often the same individuals. The first hospitals were in monasteries, founded by physicians who were usually monks. Today, many cultures throughout the world continue to regard their healers as a source for guidance in matters of faith and wellness. In the West, religion and medicine were fused until the end of the Middle Ages in the mid-1400s. Philosophers such as Descartes (1596–1650), Locke (1632–1704), and Hume (1711–1766) promoted the scientific basis of knowledge, believing that truth could only be realized through the examination of empirical data and the rational, scientific method. Centuries later, Western societies continue to experience the consequences of this split between religion and medicine. Western physicians are educated to think primarily in terms of what can be empirically proven in the laboratory. Discussions of spirituality and religion are considered by many physicians to be "off limits," with such discussion belonging to spiritual or religious leaders. In the past, when arguments arose between religion and medicine, religion usually did not fare well. Thus, many religious leaders today are cautious about what science is beginning to say about their faith.

Research has shown that religious practices such as worship attendance and prayer have significant health and survival implications. People's religiousness not only influences healthy behaviors but also influences how individuals view and define illness. A study of elderly inpatients found that one-third of those surveyed believed that sickness was a punishment from God, and nearly four-fifths felt that good health was a blessing from God. A study of hospitalized psychiatric patients found that nearly half of those surveyed believed that leading a moral life could protect against illness, and almost three-quarters attributed their illness to a sin against God. Some religions stress prayer as the way to mobilize self-healing and believe that biomedical interventions, such as surgery or blood transfusions, are harmful or sinful.

In some situations, religion may have a negative impact on people's lives. Religious participation can lead to more, not fewer, problems when unscrupulous leaders coerce or manipulate others to give up all personal autonomy. Problems also can occur when religion fosters excessive guilt or shame or encourages people to avoid dealing with life's problems. Some religious groups urge their members to avoid all conventional medical care, which can lead to life-threatening situations.

How Does Spiritual Healing Work?

No one really knows how praying for others works. Skeptics say it cannot happen, because no accepted scientific theory explains it. In the development of theories, however, empirical facts often lead to the development of an explanatory theory. For example, it was well known that penicillin worked before anyone discovered how it worked. The debate has now shifted from whether prayer works to how prayer works.

Prayer: Much More Than a Chat with God

Prayer is most often defined simply as a form of communication and fellowship with the Deity or Creator. The universality of prayer is evidenced in all cultures having some form of prayer. Prayer has been and continues to be used in times of difficulty and illness even in the most secular societies. A common image of prayer in the United States is something like this: "Prayer is talking aloud to yourself, to a white, male, cosmic parent figure, who prefers to be addressed in English." This cultural view of prayer fails to encompass how prayer is regarded by many people through-out the world. For some, prayer is more a state of being than of doing; for others, prayer is silence rather than words; for some, prayer is a thought or a desire of the heart; others pray to a female Goddess or a Divine Being who looks like they do. Buddhists do not believe in a personal God as creator and ruler of the world. Yet prayers, offered to the universe, are central to the Buddhist tradition. Prayer may be simply being still and knowing that God is God.

Prayer is part of many religious traditions and rituals and may be individual or communal, public or private. Dr. Larry Dossey, who is a private practicing physician and the leading researcher and practitioner studying the integration of spirituality and western medicine, provides a broad definition of prayer: "Prayer is communica-tion with the Absolute. This definition is inclusive, not exclusive; it affirms religious tolerance; and it invites people to define for themselves what 'communication' is, and who or what 'the Absolute' may be." According to a Sufi saying, prayer is when you talk to God and meditation is when God talks to you. In this definition, meditation is thought of as passive and receptive and prayer as active and engaging. The boundaries between meditation and prayer, however, are often blurred.

Dossey has proposed that prayer is "nonlocal," an idea derived from the field of quantum physics. The word local means that something is present in the here and now; each of us exists here and not somewhere else, and now and not at some other time. The word nonlocal means that something is not confined by place or time. All the major theistic (belief in a personal God as creator) religions agree on the nonlocal nature of God; that God is everywhere, is not confined by space and location, and exists throughout time. According to the concept of nonlocality, consciousness cannot be localized or confined to one's brain or body, nor can it be confined to the present moment. Consciousness is basic to the universe, perhaps similar to matter and energy. According to this theory, neither energy nor information travels from one mind to another, because the two minds are not separate but rather interconnected and omniscient. Dossey has proposed that consciousness-mediated events such as prayer, telepathy, precognition, and clairvoyance may be explainable as developments continue in quantum physics. As in any new theory, the nonlocal theory raises more questions than it answers. Evidence exists that prayer works, even though the exact mechanism is unknown at this time.

The Universality of Faith

Throughout history and around the world, people have called upon a Divine Being to sustain them. People are nourished by life-affirming beliefs and philosophies. They meditate and say prayers that elicit physiological calm and a sense of peacefulness, both contributing to longer survival. Benson believes that a genetic blueprint makes believing in the Great Mystery part of people's nature. Through the process of natural selection, mutating genes retain the impulses of faith, hope, and love, and faith is a natural physiologic reaction to the threats to mortality everyone faces. Benson goes on to say that "according to my investigations, it does not matter which God you worship, nor which theology you adopt as your own. Spiritual life, in general, is very healthy."

Illness as a Spiritual Crisis

Serious illness presents a spiritual crisis. As long as people are well, they maintain their autonomy and their ability to function at home, work, or school. Their feelings of self-worth are supported as they find meaning and purpose in their many activities. Once serious illness occurs, some of these things change. Ill people may have to depend on others for personal care and experience other radical lifestyle changes. Body concept changes may threaten self-esteem. In these situations, most people are forced to reevaluate life's meaning and purpose. Religious people draw heavily on their resources of faith to see them through difficult situations like serious illness. According to a number of studies, religiously involved individuals suffer less death anxiety than do non-religious people. Highly religious people have the least fear of death and the strongest belief in an afterlife. Even people with terminal illness may experience a profound sense of psychological and spiritual well-being and wholeness as they grapple with imminent death.

The Twelve Remedies

Numerous studies demonstrate that religious involvement promotes health. It appears at this time that a number of religious "ingredients" promote health and well-being (see the list in Table 22.1, "Twelve Religious Remedies"). Although some may be found in nonreligious settings, they are more commonly found operating together in religious organizations.

Twelve Religious Remedies

Relaxation response

Healthful living

Aesthetics of worship

Whole-being worship

Confession and absolution

Support network

Shared beliefs

Ritual

Purpose in life

Turning over to a Higher Power

Positive expectations

Love for self and others

The first remedy is the relaxation response, which can be evoked with meditation and prayer. The relaxation response buffers stress by clearing the mind and freeing the body from everyday tension. Practiced regularly, the relaxation response decreases heart rate, lowers metabolic rate, decreases respirations, and slows brain waves. In addition, it enhances measures of immunity. Most worship services provide time for silent prayer or meditation as well as help people take time out from busy schedules. With regular practice of the relaxation response, people report experiencing an increase in spirituality. They often describe the presence of an energy—a power, or God—that is beyond themselves. Those who feel this presence often experience the greatest medical benefits.

The second remedy is one of healthful living. Some religious groups actively promote a healthy lifestyle as part of their doctrine. Religious proscriptions may include dietary moderation, rules about sexual behavior, and regulations regarding hygiene as well as avoidance of tobacco, alcohol, and drugs. In one survey of college students, researchers found that the more religious students avoided health-compromising behaviors and engaged in more frequent health-enhancing behaviors than those students who were less religiously involved.

Remedy number three is the aesthetics of worship, which taps into a universal appreciation for beauty. Visual symbols of faith are reassuring and calming images. Stained-glass windows, beautiful architecture, and floral arrangements all provide an experience of harmony and balance. Sacred music uses audible beauty to communicate the splendor of God. The smell of incense may evoke a deep sense of peace and quietude.

The fourth remedy is whole-being worship. Christians who sing familiar hymns, Jews who sing "Torah Ora" when the Torah scroll is presented, and Buddhists who chant their prayers all participate in whole-being worship through music. This combination of physical activity (singing), cognitive activity (reading the words), and spiritual activity (prayer through song) evokes a sense of peace. Movements such as kneeling, standing, bowing heads, folding hands, or even dancing engage people on all levels of being. As people worship with body, mind, and spirit, they go through a unifying experience that is as good for them as it feels.

Remedy number five is confession and absolution. Harboring guilty feelings can literally make people sick. In many religions, people are encouraged to confess their sins, repent, and are given assurance of forgiveness and absolution. This process allows individuals to review their mistakes, share their personal pain, and learn from and move on rather than becoming preoccupied with personal shortcomings.

The sixth remedy is one's support network—those family members and friends who offer practical help, emotional support, and spiritual encouragement in the time of need. People are social beings whose health often deteriorates when they become isolated and lonely. Lack of human companionship has been linked to depression of the immune system and a lowered production of endorphins, the neurotransmitter that produces the feeling of well-being. A 10-year study of 2,754 people found that men who volunteered regularly and had social contact with others were less likely to die than those who volunteered less and had less social contact. Another study found that elderly patients undergoing heart surgery who participated in community and social groups, like those who received comfort from their religious beliefs, were three times more likely to survive. But those who participated in both social activities and received comfort from their religious faith were 10 times more likely to survive.

Interaction with others can help people transform their attitudes and emotions, which magnifies the effect of self-healing and health enhancement efforts. Religious organizations often provide many opportunities for social interaction from religious services to sacred study groups, to youth, women's, and men's groups, and to community outreach groups. This group interaction can provide a number of healing benefits by offering a sense of partnership, helping with coping, creating a sense of community and safety, encouraging a cooperative approach to problem solving, helping to change behaviors and thoughts, supporting taking control, and encouraging personal action.

Remedy number seven is shared beliefs. Most people prefer to associate with individuals who share similar beliefs and points of view. Great things can be achieved when groups are unified around common values. Religious traditions are opportunities for people to share common beliefs. Individuals who feel they are part of a group find they are not alone and gain strength from the power of shared beliefs. Participation in regular worship not only helps people feel connected and helps them rise above their differences, but it also is an antidote to the alienation often prevalent in Western society.

The eighth remedy is ritual. Ceremony and ritual are ways of creating sacred space and time, when normal ways of relating are put aside and people can listen and pray with an open heart to their Divine Being. Religious ritual is a powerful healing mechanism that has soothing and calming effects. Rituals provide people a link with tradition and give them a sense of security.

The ninth remedy is that of finding a purpose in life. People's search for meaning is held by many to be the primary motivation in their lives. This search for meaning becomes more intense during periods of illness as people struggle with age-old questions such as: Why me? Why now? Did I do something to deserve this? Religion and worship attendance provide a framework of meaning, a sense of purpose in life, and a meaningful interpretation for difficult times. People who are dying often seem to arrive at a sense of what life's purpose is. As they tell it, the purpose of life is to grow in wisdom and to learn to love better. They discover that health is not an end but rather a means. In other words, health enables people to serve a purpose in life, but health is not the purpose in life.

Remedy number ten is turning one's life over to the Great Mystery or God. It is an acknowledgment that no one has total control over her or his life. Religion provides an avenue for asking for guidance, intervention, and strength. Faith in a God who is loving and caring provides comfort for those going through difficult times. Worship services often leave people feeling less burdened and anxious, as well as more peaceful.

The eleventh remedy is that of positive expectations. During a time of illness or distress, religion often provides a sense of hope and the strength to endure what has happened. The expectancy of help from the Divine Source works similarly, as does the expectancy of help from a medication, procedure, or caregiver. Various holy writings promise health and healing to the faithful, and researchers are beginning to document the effect of this expectation on the outcome of disease.

The twelfth, and last, remedy is love for self and others. All religions focus on loving God and other people. This love includes helping others, strangers as well as family and friends. When people love and help others, they often experience better health than those who do not.

These 12 religious remedies can be found outside of religious organizations. Frequent religious participation, however, provides many of these remedies in one context. Research is demonstrating that religious participation is an important factor in the prevention of disease, achievement of well-being, healing from illness, and extension of life span. One mystery that remains, however, is why some people are cured and others are not. One can be very spiritual and still get sick and die. It must be remembered that religious participation and spirituality are no guarantee for physical health. Failure to recognize this basic reality can result in inappropriate self-blame.

How Do I Begin Taking a Spiritual Approach to My Health?

Some people seek out nurses, doctors, counselors, and therapists who focus on spiritual concerns as well as physical and emotional concerns. This focus is especially helpful for those who are dealing with issues related to meaning and purpose in life. Alternatively, people may seek the help of a religious leader who includes healing practices in her or his religious practice. Faith healing has not been scientifically proven but remains a popular option for many. Some people go to specific places for healing. The Catholic Church has documented 36 "miracles" at Lourdes, for example. A variety of spiritually focused healing groups are also available. People with addictive disorders benefit from 12-step programs, which rely on both group support and the specific invocation of a Higher Power.

Two different types of prayer are directed and nondirected. In directed prayer, the praying person asks for a specific outcome, such as for the cancer to go away or for the baby to be born healthy. In contrast, in nondirected prayer, no specific outcome is asked. The praying person simply asks for the best thing to occur in a given situation. Studies show that both approaches are effective in promoting health.

Prayer can also be described according to form. Colloquial prayer is an informal talk with God, as if one were talking to a good friend. Petitional prayer or intercessory prayer is asking God for things for oneself or others. The focus is on what God can provide. Intercessory prayer is often called "distant" prayer, because the person being prayed for is often remote from the person who is praying. This form of prayer is of current interest to researchers. Ritual prayer is the use of formal prayers or rituals such as prayers from a prayer book or in the Jewish siddur, or the Catholic practice of saying the rosary. Meditative prayer, also known as contemplative prayer, is similar to meditation and is a process of focusing the mind on an aspect of God for a period of time.

Surveys by *USA Today Weekend* and *Time* indicate that nearly two out of three Americans would like their physicians to address spiritual issues and to pray with them, if they so request. In a study of people who were hospitalized, more than 75% believed that their physician should address spiritual issues as a part of their medical care. Not only did they want them to discuss these issues, but nearly half wanted their physician to pray with them. Unfortunately, these same clients reported that spirituality and religion were hardly ever addressed, less than 1% of the time, as part of their medical care.

Of course, some nurses and physicians do incorporate faith and prayer into their care. Dr. Alijani, a faculty member at Georgetown University Medical School and a well-known surgeon, believes that faith plays a significant role in his patient's well-being. He sees prayer as the literal lifeline between health and spirituality: "Just as my body needs water, carbohydrates, protein, and lipids, my mind needs Allah, and the only way to receive Allah is to pray."

Why is it that some doctors and nurses do not incorporate faith and prayer into their professional practice? Some are unaware of the research data regarding the faith factor. That situation is beginning to change as schools of nursing develop courses to teach students about the faith-health connection. Some have been told specifically that they are not to mix nursing and faith. This recommendation was made out of a concern that they might blur the professional-personal boundaries and cause harm to patients.

Health care practitioners are not meant to replace clergy. The roles are distinct. Although many patients may want their spiritual needs addressed by nurses and physicians, others do not, preferring to have these issues addressed by clergy. The practitioner needs to take into account, however, where and how the client's belief enters into the healing process. Nor should health care practitioners be forced against their wishes into participating in client's religious practices. In the best of worlds, health care professionals and clergy work closely together to provide meaningful holistic care.

TRY IT YOURSELF: INCORPORATING THE BENEFITS OF PRAYER

- If you are ill, ask specifically for people's prayers for healing. It may involve clergy, members of a congregation, adding your name to a prayer list, or asking family and friends to pray for you on a regular basis.
- Pray for your own healing.
- Seek out healing services. Many churches and synagogues offer opportunities to participate in a prayer service or healing service.
- Pray persistently. Keep praying regardless of apparent results. Continuing prayer is an expression of faith and hope.
- Pray for others who are suffering.

Prayer as an Act of Gratitude

You may also want to take time out to count your blessings and say "thanks" for the good things in life. Paying attention to what you already have and what is going right in your life helps alleviate stress, anxiety, and depression. An act of gratitude often restores a sense of balance and perspective.

- Remember to say "thank you." Make it a habit whenever someone helps you out, gives you a compliment, or gives you a gift.
- Create rituals of thanks; for example, saying grace before meals or daily prayers. Practice them until they become a habit.
- Every night before you go to bed, make a list of five things you are grateful for. It will help take the focus off the stresses in your life.
- Take the time to give back. Look for opportunities to help others and recycle the good fortune you have in your life.
- Once a day, strike a grateful pose. It could be kneeling in prayer or standing with your arms extended joyfully to the sky.
- Take 10 minutes each day to be grateful. Go outside into nature, meditate, or pray. Whatever you do, take the time to appreciate all that you have right now.

FAITH AND PRAYER ASSESSMENT

- What does your faith mean to you? Has it changed during your illness?

- What is the importance of this faith in your daily life?

- Do your beliefs influence the way you think about your health or look at your illness?

- How important is your religious identification? Do you belong to an organized group?

- List your religious practices, such as worship, prayer, or meditation.

- What is the role of prayer in your life?

- How are your prayers answered?

PROJECTING LOVE

1. Visualize someone for whom you have loving feelings. Let the love you feel surround your whole body inside and out. Concentrate on these feelings and project them to this person.

2. Next, visualize someone toward whom you have warm feelings that are not as strong as for the first person. As you focus, send these feelings of love and appreciation to that person.

3. Next, visualize someone toward whom you have neutral feelings, nothing strong either way. As you focus on the person, bring the same intensity of love and appreciation you felt for the first two people to the third. Send these feelings to that person.

4. Now visualize someone you have some difficulty with, perhaps whom you dislike but not very intensely. Bring to this person the same feelings of love and appreciation.

5. Finally, visualize someone you have a strong dislike for, and again, as you focus on this person, bring the same degree of love and appreciation you felt for the others. It may be helpful to focus on the person's heart as you do this exercise. Send these feelings to that person.

THE ABSOLUTE MINIMUM

- While no one knows for sure how spiritual healing works, the evidence is plentiful that is does.

- It's theorized that the contemplative, ritual practices fostered by religious observance combine to create a healing effect that's larger than the combination of the individual practices.

- The benefits of spiritual healing can be obtained by maintaining an attitude of reverence and gratitude toward the universe, whether part of a religious orthodoxy or not.

RESOURCES

- Common Boundary

  www.commonboundary.org

- Fellowship in Prayer, Inc.

  www.fip.org

- The Interface Between Medicine and Religion, John Templeton Foundation

  www.templeton.org

- Shalem Institute for Spiritual Formation

  www.shalem.org

PART VII

OTHER THERAPIES

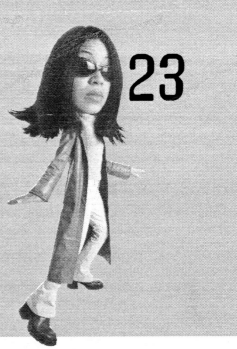

23

BIOELECTROMAGNETICS

Bioelectromagnetics (BEM) is the emerging science that studies how living organisms interact with electromagnetic (EM) fields. What underlies all of biochemistry is electromagnetism, a form of energy. Quantum physics has demonstrated that what people see as solid matter, be that a person or an object, is actually 99.9999 percent empty space filled with energy. Everything is, in fact, energy vibrating at different rates.

The earth is 85 percent crystal. Its crust is largely silicon and oxygen, combined with aluminum, iron, calcium, sodium, potassium, and magnesium. From these chemicals come a wide variety of crystal colors, shapes, sizes, and hardness. Different crystals are formed under varying conditions of temperature, pressure, space, and time. Diamonds, for example, are found only at a few locations in the world because the exact conditions for their formation are relatively rare.

Crystals are solid minerals with a symmetrical internal atomic structure and can be classified according to their external appearance: cubic, tetragonal, hexagonal, trigonal, orthorhombic, monoclinic, and triclinic. The most desirable crystals are called precious or semiprecious gemstones such as diamonds, amethyst, aquamarine, rose quartz, opal, topaz, and turquoise. Crystal healing works on the principle that every animal, plant, and mineral has an electromagnetic field that enables organic beings and inorganic objects, such as crystals, to communicate and interact as part of a single, unified energy system. Imitation or synthetic gemstones are material made to look like a gem but have a different chemical structure and physical properties. An example would be blue glass cut to imitate sapphire. As such, synthetic crystals will not display the same electromagnetic properties as natural crystals.

What Is Bioelectromagnetics?

In the 18th century, Guigi Galvani, an Italian physician conducted experiments on frog muscle to demonstrate that bioelectricity exists within living tissue. Shortly after that, Alessandro Volta, a physicist, found that animal tissue was not needed to produce a current and went on to invent the electric battery in 1800. Michael Faraday, a British chemist, became the greatest experimentalist in electricity and magnetism of the 19th century, produced the first electric motor, and succeeded in showing that a magnet could induce electricity. From this early work came many devices for the diagnosis and treatment of disease, including many that are in use today.

In the late 1950s in Japan, doctors began to see a new syndrome of low energy, insomnia, and generalized aches and pains. After extensive research it was discovered that these complaints came from people who spent large amounts of time in metal buildings and were thus shielded from the earth's natural magnetic field. The disorder was labeled "magnetic field deficiency syndrome," and symptoms were alleviated by the external application of magnetic fields to the patients' bodies. Today, magnetic healing continues to be a significant part of mainstream medicine in Japan.

Similarly, early Russian cosmonauts who spent more than a year in space were amazed to find that they had lost nearly 80% of their bone density. As a result, spacecrafts were designed to include strong artificial magnetic fields on board to avoid this problem. Both of these examples illustrate how magnetic fields are essential to good health and well-being.

Throughout the ages, crystals have been a part of cultural development. Early people used crystals to make tools and weapons and to generate a spark to make fire. Crystals, or gemstones, were also portable forms of wealth and status. The oldest examples of jewelry made of gold, silver, and semi-precious stones were found in the tomb of Queen Puabi at Ur, which dates back to 3000 BC. Early Egyptians were the first to develop cosmetics, and to highlight their eyes with powdered malachite (green) and lapis lazuli (blue). Gemstones were worn as amulets, objects believed to bring good luck, protect against evil, and ensure safe travel after death into the next life. The contemporary custom of wearing birthstones is a reflection of this history. Native Americans believed quartz crystals to be the home of supernatural forces that would bring good luck to their hunting trips. The first known reference to the healing power of certain crystals comes from an Egyptian papyrus from 1600 BC. It gave directions for curative use, such as placing crystals on various areas of the body and grinding them up and mixing with a liquid for internal consumption.

Geomagnetic Field

Every atom and cell of the body is a small magnetic field that radiates out into space, decreasing in strength with distance and ultimately becoming lost in the jumble of other magnetic fields. Like the human body, the earth radiates an energy field outwardly, called the geomagnetic field. This energy originates in the earth's core and radiates out beyond the atmosphere, stimulating and protecting all of life on earth. Animals are attuned to the geomagnetic field and can sense subtle changes in it. For example, dogs, horses, and cattle often become agitated just before an earthquake.

note

Migrating birds or fish returning to their spawning grounds navigate over great distances with the help of magnetic field receptors in their brains. It is believed that they tune in to the magnetic field of the earth to determine location and direction.

A magnetic field is like a generator, generating internal energy that can penetrate the body as if it were air. A strong magnet held on one side of the hand can easily deflect a compass needle on the other side of the same hand. As the magnetic field penetrates the body, it causes one's atomic particles to fly around faster and interact with more force.

Subtle changes occur in the strength of the geomagnetic field with the time of day. The daytime side of the planet—that side facing the sun—always has a slightly weaker field, because the energy coming out of the earth is being "pushed" back and compressed by the radiation from the sun. Thus, the magnetic field passing through the human body is stronger on the nighttime side, away from the sun. Chemical reactions, the healing process, and other cellular activities accelerate in the presence of a stronger field, and thus they are improved slightly at night because of the stronger field.

Like a giant mirror, the moon reflects radiation from the sun toward the earth, thus affecting the earth's energy field. The full moon and the new moon are opposite in their effect on the geomagnetic field. The greatest amount of solar radiation is reflected toward the earth during a full moon, which pushes back and compresses the earth's energy, resulting in a weaker magnetic field than during a new moon. Study results have been mixed as to the effect on human behavior, but a study done throughout the calendar year 1993 in Las Vegas found that the full moon was associated with a rise in psychotic behavior, an increase in suicide rates, and an abrupt increase in crisis calls to "911."

A stronger magnetic field is more conducive to sleep, which makes sleep at night more refreshing and healing than sleep in the daytime. In addition, the sun "agitates" the earth's field with sunspot activity. These intense magnetic explosions on the sun spray additional radiation on the earth, in turn disturbing the geomagnetic field. During these periods of geomagnetic disturbance, higher admission rates to psychiatric facilities and higher rates of violence are characteristic. On the other hand, when the earth's magnetic field is most quiet, more paranormal experiences like mental telepathy, clairvoyance, and precognition take place.

Endogenous Magnetic Fields

Endogenous magnetic fields are those produced within the body. This electrical activity demonstrates patterns that provide medically useful information. EKGs and EEGs, for example, provide information about the endogenous magnetic fields of the heart and brain and are diagnostic in any number of conditions.

Like other kinds of magnetic fields, the human energy field is strongest at its source and fades with distance. Another name for this energy field is "aura" and it is the field that surrounds the body as far as the outstretched arms and from head to toe. The human energy field is both an information center and a highly sensitive perceptual system that transmits and receives messages as people interact with their surrounding environment. Patterns of circulation of energy within the body include the meridian system and the chakras. Virtually every alternative healing therapy has a way of interpreting these subtle energy fields.

Recent research has uncovered a form of endogenous radiation, an extremely low-level light known as biophoton emission. It is believed that biophoton emission may be important in gene expression, membrane transport, and bioregulation. Externally applied energy fields may alter biophoton emission to the benefit or detriment of the organism. This, as well as other endogenous fields of the body may prove to be involved in energetic therapies such as Therapeutic Touch.

Exogenous Magnetic Fields

Exogenous magnetic fields are those produced by sources outside the body and can be classified as either artificial or natural. Artificial exogenous fields are created by the presence of power lines, transformers, appliances, radio transmitters, and medical devices. Some of these may be harmful, such as those fields emitted by power lines, which are linked to an increased risk of childhood leukemia. Artificial electromagnetic fields are unpolarized. Their behavior is chaotic and disordered as they pass through the body's cells. This chaotic nature disturbs the endogenous magnetic fields, resulting in damage to the body's tissues.

The earth's geomagnetic field is one example of a natural exogenous field. Another example is moving water. When you are at the beach, on river banks, beside waterfalls, or even walking outside after a powerful rainstorm, you often experience feelings of relaxation and peace. While these feelings may be attributed to the psychological cues from these environments, they also have an energetic basis. When water moves or flows, it releases negative ions into the air. When people are surrounded by negative ions, they seem to balance their energy fields.

Resonance

Another principle, related to electromagnetics, is resonance, which is simply defined as sympathetic vibration. For example, when a tuning fork turned to note A is sounded near a piano or guitar, any string that is tuned to that same tone will pick up the vibration and begin to move, while the other strings will not. Crystals possess electromagnetic properties and are capable of resonating in harmony with another form. It is believed that when the body's natural frequencies become unbalanced, people experience dis-ease. The resonance of crystals is believed to harmonize and balance the body's frequencies back to optimum, healthy levels. The disrupted field (the ill person) receives energy from the stronger field (the crystal) until the two find their own balance and resonate in harmony. At the current time, however, no explanations for crystal healing fit within known scientific facts.

SOME APPLICATIONS OF BIOELECTROMAGNETICS

- **Transcultaneous electrical nerve stimulation (TENS)**—Used for pain relief

- **Transcranial electrostimulation (TCES)**—Used to reduce symptoms of depression, anxiety, and insomnia; may be effective in drug dependence

- **Neuromagnetic stimulation**—Used in place of electro-convulsive therapy in certain types of mood disorders; used in diagnostic nerve conduction studies

- **Electromyography**—Used to diagnose and treat carpal tunnel syndrome and other movement disorders

- **Electroencephalography**—Along with EEG biofeedback, used to treat attention deficit disorder, learning disabilities, stroke, and alcoholism

- **Electroretinography**— Noninvasive monitoring of rapid eye movement sleep

- **Low energy emission therapy**—Used to treat insomnia and hypertension

How Does Bioelectromagnetics Work?

Magnetic and crystal healing work best in combination with other healing methods and should be considered as adjunct treatments to conventional medicine. Magnetic and crystal healing should not be used alone for any major disease or medical condition.

Magnetic Therapies: They're Very Attractive

Being immersed in a field of negative ions seems to balance people's energy and relieve pain. Physicians specializing in orthopedics and sports medicine have been recommending magnets since 1993. Athletic performance is enhanced and risk of serious injury is decreased when magnets are used to warm up muscles and joints. People wear magnets on their wrists, elbows, and knees for joint pain or on their heads for headaches. Magnets are used to speed the healing of wounds. Though not recognized as medical devices by the Food and Drug Administration, magnets have been widely used in Asia for years. Blood cells, believed to have tiny positive charges at one end and negative charges at the other end, respond to the pull of magnets, thus increasing blood flow to the area. The increased blood flow brings in more healing nutrients and carries off toxins. Magnets appear to block pain by altering the electro-magnetic balance between negatively charged and positively charged ions in the nerve pathways that carry pain messages. The magnets used are about

5–10 times as strong as refrigerator door magnets and cost between $12 and $28 a pair depending on the size.

A few contraindications for magnetic therapy need to be observed. Until further research is conducted, pregnant women should not wear magnets over the abdominal area. Magnets should not be used by anyone wearing a pacemaker, defibrillator, or other implanted electrical device. Magnets decrease the stickiness of platelets, which contributes to increased bleeding. For that reason, they should not be used with people on anticoagulants or who have an actively bleeding wound.

Crystal Healing: A Therapeutic Wavelength

Crystal healing is based on tuning in to the natural vibrations of a mineral from the earth, which has infused it with its energies. For this reason, neither imitation nor synthetic crystals are suitable for healing. In electrocrystal therapy, the body is initially scanned with a specially adapted video camera that relays a colored picture of the auric field onto a computer screen. The therapist marks those areas where the color of the aura is inappropriate, indicating stress or dysfunction. Electrocrystal therapy uses quartz crystals in saline solution that are enclosed in a sealed, glass electrode connected to a battery. Up to five electrodes are placed against the affected area or over a chakra point. The crystals are electrically stimulated, which amplifies their natural healing vibrations until they vibrate and resonate at a desired frequency. This treatment is thought to bring the endogenous fields back to a harmonious state.

Crystal cards, created to be worn on the body, were developed as a result of the NASA space program. Astronauts travel into space with a number of pyramid-shaped quartz crystals, electronically charged to vibrate at the frequency of the earth's geomagnetic field, to combat the negative effects of spending time outside the earth's magnetic field. The crystal cards sold in stores contain a number of tiny corundum crystals that are electrochemically etched with hydrochloric acid. The acid changes the form of the crystals, which produces beneficial negative ions and harmonizes cellular activity.

Electronic gem therapy blends modern technology with traditional Ayurvedic medicine by combining gemstones or crystals, colored light, and electronic amplification. Depending on the condition, patients either require cooling gems such as emerald, topaz, or carnelian or warming gems such as ruby, chrysoberyl, or citrine. During treatment the gemstone is electronically vibrated at a frequency set for a specific condition. The energy from the gemstone is focused via special-colored lamps called gem transducers onto the part of the body requiring treatment. It is believed the treatment provides additional energy needed to bring about self-healing. The seven chakras are assigned different gemstones corresponding to their vibratory rates. In crystal bodywork, people place crystals on the chakras as they meditate.

CRYSTALS, GEMSTONES, AND CHAKRAS

Root Chakra

Agate, bloodstone, tiger's eye, hematite

Sexual Chakra

Moonstone, tiger's eye, citrine, carnelian

Solar Plexus Chakra

Citrine, rose quartz, aventurine quartz, malachite

Heart Chakra

Jade, aventurine quartz, watermelon tourmaline, rose quartz

Throat Chakra

Aquamarine, lapis lazuli, turquoise, celestite

Third Eye Chakra

Amethyst, fluorite, lapis lazuli, sodalite

Crown Chakra

Amethyst, celestite, jade, rock crystal (clear quartz)

Getting Started with Bioelectromagnetic Healing

While the magnetic fields in the earth and our bodies are both unavoidable and free, you must create and work with a third field to tap their healing potential. This section explores how to obtain and use crystals and magnets for this purpose.

Choosing a Crystal

Many people use crystals in combination with other healing methods. Some people choose crystals intuitively, while others select crystals on the basis of therapeutic qualities. The following questions can help you determine which crystal is "right" for you:

■ What do you want the crystal for—healing, meditation, energizing your environment, as a focus for visualization, or for decoration?

■ Which crystals are most appealing—geometrically shaped, such as clear quartz, or "massive," such as rose quartz?

■ Which colors are appealing to you—pale or deep shades? Do you prefer clear or opaque?

■ What size crystal are you looking for?

■ Do you prefer cut and polished crystals or ones that are completely natural?

■ How much are you prepared to spend?

Meditating with Your Crystal

Members of the quartz family, such as clear quartz, amethyst, and rose quartz, are the crystals used most frequently in healing. Amethyst is the "stone of meditation," creating a state of enhanced spirituality and contentment. Clear quartz represents the clarity of mind that people hope to achieve through meditation. Maintaining a focus on a crystal helps quiet thoughts during meditation. Hold the crystal or place it in front of you on the floor or on a small table. Some people take three similar crystals and position them in an equilateral triangle, forming a charged energy field in which to sit. Half-close your eyes and gaze at the crystal, concentrating on its color, shape, and size during your meditation. As you come out of the meditative state, you should continue to focus on the crystal and open your eyes gradually.

People who are experiencing illness or disease may find that crystal imagery improves the healing process. You can follow the Pink Bubble guided imagery technique given in Chapter 16, "Meditation," substituting your crystal for the pink bubble:

■ Assume your meditative position and focus on the crystal in front of you.

■ Close your eyes, while continuing to visualize the crystal.

■ Allow this image of the crystal to become bigger and bigger until it completely surrounds you.

■ Imagine that you are at the center of the crystal.

■ Notice how you have become one with the crystal.

■ Image the illness or disease leaving your body as you become one with the crystal.

■ Consider how it feels to share the same perfection and clarity as the crystal. Be aware that you are whole and complete as you are one with the crystal.

■ Contemplate how the crystal forms a protective shield around you so that you are totally safe and secure.

■ When you sense that your inner journey is completed, begin to separate yourself from the crystal.

■ Reduce the crystal to its normal size.

■ Fade this picture from your mind, open your eyes, and take a few deep breaths to bring yourself back into the here and now.

■ Be aware of any thoughts, feelings, or emotions that come to you.

Trying Magnetic Therapies

Awareness of magnetic healing is gaining credibility in the United States and is being applied by increasing numbers of conventional as well as alternative health-care practitioners as an adjunctive therapy. Increasing numbers of people are sleeping on magnetic beds at night and wearing small magnets during the day for pain relief, greater energy, and healing.

Some controversy surrounds the issue of when to use the north, or negative pole, and when to use the south, or positive pole. Some people believe that the north pole of a magnet enhances healing and health while the south pole exacerbates disease. Practitioners in Japan and Russia believe no strong evidence supports the use of one pole over the other but rather that the entirety of the magnet is doing the healing.

The effectiveness of magnetic treatment depends on the number of magnets used and their strength, thickness, and spacing. Magnets vary in strength and those used for healing purposes are generally between 1,000 and 5,000 gauss. In general, healing magnets are unipolar and are either circular or rectangular. Several can be stacked for increased gauss strength and, therefore, greater effectiveness: the thicker the magnet, the greater the depth of penetration. The problem with this is that, with increasing thickness, the magnet becomes more uncomfortable to wear. Most people wear magnets between one-fourth and three-eighths of an inch thick. In general, the magnet should be larger than the size of the area being treated. Patients who are treating finger joints for arthritis will use a small magnet, while those who are treating the lower back will apply a much larger magnet.

The most common use of magnetic therapy is in pain treatment, with reports of successful treatment in arthritis, rheumatism, fibromyalgia, back pain, headaches, muscle sprains and strains, joint pain, tendonitis, shoulder pain, carpal tunnel syndrome, and torn ligaments. A magnetic field can also function like an antibiotic by lowering acidity, creating a hostile environment for microorganisms. A magnetic field applied to the head has a sedating effect by stimulating the hormone melatonin. Biomagnetic therapy increases general well-being by enhancing energy through cell repolarization. Many professional athletes revitalize their bodies by sleeping on a magnetic mattress pad. Some even participate in their sport with dozens of magnets taped to their bodies.

Magnetic therapy may be one of the most effective methods for achieving relief from arthritis, especially in the hands and feet. People with carpal tunnel syndrome can apply magnets to the front and back of the wrist to help control symptoms. Individuals diagnosed with fibromyalgia can sleep on a magnetic mattress pad and use a magnetic pillow, as well as using magnets over the painful areas during the day. Magnetic insoles increase circulation and help conditions such as numbness, burning, aches, restlessness, and leg cramps. People with asthma and bronchitis may find that wearing a strong neodymium magnet over the chest and at an equal level on the back will help return breathing to a normal state. For minor burns, people can place a magnet over the site of injury to speed up the healing and reduce the pain.

It is unclear at this time whether you should wear the magnets full time or intermittently, though researchers are studying this and other issues of magnetic therapy. Until a consensus emerges, you should experiment with time periods that seem most effective. As scientific and clinical understanding increases, we will be able to provide greater knowledge about how to manipulate magnets for the best effects.

TRY IT YOURSELF: ABSORBING EARTH ENERGY

Find a grassy, open area that is in its relatively natural state. You may choose to use a blanket or not. Lie face down with your arms and legs extended in a spreading out fashion. Notice that all your chakras are in direct contact with the earth. Visualize an exchange of energy as you release to the earth, with each out-breath, any stress or negativity you have been carrying. With each in-breath, imagine that your chakras are receiving fresh, balanced, healing energy from the earth. Do this relaxation breathing for at least 20 minutes. You should feel yourself in a pleasant and refreshed state.

THE ABSOLUTE MINIMUM

- Bioelectromagnetic therapies seek to influence health and well-being by modifying the electromagnetic fields created by the earth, our bodies, and special crystals and magnets used in the healing process.

- While no consensus exists on how, or even whether, bioelectromagnetic therapies work, the effects have achieved greater acceptance in other countries, and are being studied by U.S. government agencies like the NIH and NASA.

- Adding crystals and therapeutic magnets to existing practices of meditation and healthful living is at worst harmless, and at best a way to tap the healing forces of the entire planet.

RESOURCES

- *Subtle Energy.* W. Collinge, 1998, Warner Books, New York.

- *The Book of Crystal Healing.* L. Simpson, 1997, Sterling Publishing, New York.

- Center for Specific Cancer Therapy

  www.csct.com

- International Society for the Study of Subtle Energies and Energy Medicine (ISSSEEM)

  www.issseem.org

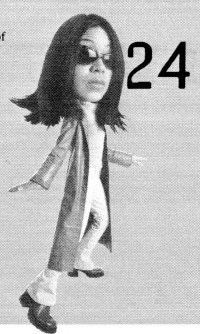

24

Detoxifying Therapies

Many cultures and religions, past and present, consider people or things they find evil or unhealthy to be "unclean" and most have developed rituals of purification to correct this. In Western cultures, some people are currently fascinated with the concept of detoxification, the belief that physical impurities and toxins must be cleared from the body to achieve better health, in most cases using our most ancient and basic therapeutic substance: water. This chapter provides an overview of several ways people use water to clean their bodies inside and out: hydrotherapy, colonics, and chelation therapy.

Hydrotherapy: A Nice, Hot Bath

Water has been a part of healing practices from ancient times and great healing powers have been attributed to it as seen in phrases like "healing waters" and the "fountain of youth." The Romans built bathhouses throughout their empire. Saunas have been popular in Scandinavian countries for many years and have risen in popularity in the United States in the latter half of the 20th century. In Europe and the United States, people go to spas that have been built around the mineral waters of natural hot springs for periods of rest and rejuvenation . Today, hydrotherapy, or water-based therapy, is used to treat wounds, injuries, and burns, to promote physical rehabilitation, and to manage stress

The use of water as a healing treatment is known as hydrotherapy. Nurses, chiropractors, physical therapists, naturopaths, massage therapists, yoga masters, and conventional physicians incorporate various forms of hydrotherapy in their professional practice. Programs of study in each discipline cover the use of hydrotherapy techniques that are appropriate for the particular professional practice.

Hydrotherapy, the use of hot and cold moisture in the form of solid, liquid, or gas, makes use of the body's response to heat and cold. The primary effect of both heat and cold is stimulation. The secondary effects of heat are drowsiness, sedation, and relaxed muscles. Heat also dilates blood vessels, increasing the circulation to the area being heated. The secondary effects of cold are invigoration and restoration. Cold constricts blood vessels, reducing circulation to that area of the body. Hydrotherapy is used to decrease pain, decrease fever, reduce swelling, lessen cramps, induce sleep, and improve physical and mental tone. It must be used with great care in the young and the old who have poor heat regulation and also with people experiencing a prolonged illness or fatigue.

Three basic types of hydrotherapy are compresses, bathing, and sweat baths. The general use of compresses involves towels wrung out in hot and cold water and alternately applied to the body. The intense fluctuations in temperature are believed to improve the circulation to the stomach, liver, kidneys, and intestines, thereby improving digestion and the elimination of metabolic wastes. Other examples of compresses include ice packs to reduce the swelling of sprained ankles and hot water packs for muscle pain.

Baths, as a form of hydrotherapy, involve local baths such as a foot, sitz, and full immersion baths. They may be hot or cold or alternating. Hot water, and the substances sometimes added to the water, increase blood flow to the skin, open pores, and increase sweating, all of which lead to a faster release of toxins. Warm water is often used to irrigate and cleanse wounds. Full immersion baths are used for physical rehabilitation. Exercising in water can be more effective and cause less strain to the skeleton and joints than exercise out of water.

Sweat baths are a method of detoxification that enables the body to eliminate salt, drugs, and a variety of toxins. They are typically done in a steam room or a sauna.

A process in yoga called *neti* (pronounced NAY-tee) involves various methods for cleansing the nasal passages. One method is to sniff warm water into the nostrils and spit it out of the mouth. Neti bottles are also available and are designed to pour water into one nostril, which will then come out the other nostril.

> ## caution
> Pregnant women should never use sweat bathing, as the heat may cause neural tube defects in the first trimester. Sweat baths are not recommended for people with heart disease, kidney disease, or anemia.

Colonics: A Deeper Feeling of Clean

Written documents of ancient Egypt and Greece contain references to colon therapy. For hundreds of years, nurses and physicians have advocated enemas as internal body baths. Colon therapy was introduced to the United States at the end of the 19th century, and it rapidly became popular. Healthy people used enemas to cleanse and rejuvenate themselves. Others used enemas to treat heart disease, hypertension, arthritis, depression, and various infections. In the mid-20th century, as antibiotics and other medications became available, colon therapy began to fade from popular use. In the 1980s, a resurgence of colonics took place in the United States among people who believe that their bodies are full of harmful chemicals, by-products, food residues, or accumulated intestinal waste. This desire for cleansing has created a growing market for products and treatments that claim to detoxify the body and restore it to a state of purity.

The International Association for Colon Hydrotherapy (I-ACT) is the certifying body for colon hydrotherapy training. A list of schools teaching the I-ACT syllabus, as well as names of colon therapists, is available from the association. The foundation level of education includes a 100-hour course of colon hydrotherapy training from an approved school or certified instructor as well as a 100-hour internship. In addition, students must pass a written exam. The intermediate level requirements include 500 hours of course work, a demonstration of expertise, and an intermediate exam. The instructor level requirements include 1,000 hours of training or three years of practice. In addition, teaching skills must be demonstrated.

Colonics, or colon therapy, is based on the idea that high-fat, Western diets lead to an accumulation of a thick, glue-like substance in the colon, which in turn produces toxins that lead to disease. Colonics, also called colonic irrigation or high colonics, is a procedure for washing the inner wall of the colon by filling it with water or herbal solutions and then draining it. Colonics are a technique for removing any material that may be present high in the colon and cleans the entire five feet of the colon compared to enemas, which clean only the lower 8–12 inches of the colon. Colonics, administered by a colon therapist, uses 2–6 liters of liquid at a time; the therapist then massages the colon through the abdomen, and the water is eliminated through a waste tube. The procedure is repeated over a period of 30–45 minutes, and uses more than 20 gallons of water per session.

Colon cleansing is a controversial method of detoxification, and there tends to be no middle ground in the beliefs about the usefulness of colonics. People tend to either strongly support or challenge the practice of colonics. Those who support colonics believe that toxicity can build up in the pockets of the colon through years of a diet heavy in fried foods, white flour, sugar, refined and processed foods, dairy products, carbonated beverages, and not enough fiber. The use of prescription drugs, tobacco, and alcoholic beverages are additional sources of toxicity. Substances generally used for colonics include water, coffee, herbal teas, a mild soap solution, meat broth, wheat grass juice, and barley juice. I-ACT recommends the use of colonics twice yearly as a maintenance regimen. Colonics is not recommended for people in a weakened state and those having ulcerative colitis, diverticulitis, Crohn's disease, severe hemorrhoids, or tumors of the large intestine or rectum.

Those who oppose the use of colonics believe no medical reason supports its use. It is believed that diet, water, and exercise should be enough to maintain the health of the colon. Andrew Weil states, "I have reviewed many systems of colon cleansing, including colonic irrigation (colonics) and the use of natural laxatives and herbal mixtures. If you eat a high-fiber diet, drink plenty of water, exercise, and move your bowels regularly, you shouldn't need any of them. The best way to care for the colon is to let its own natural physiological action keep it clean and in good working order." Problems that may result from colonics include enzyme imbalance, perforation of the colon, and general weakening of the body.

Chelation Therapy: No More Heavy Metal

Chelation comes from the Greek work chele or "claw." When chelation chemicals are introduced into the bloodstream, they bind, or claw, to heavy metals in the body. Ethylene diamine tetraacetic acid (EDTA) is a synthetic amino acid that readily binds to heavy metals. EDTA was synthesized in the 1940s and was originally used by the United States Navy to remove calcium from pipes and boilers. In the 1950s, EDTA was tried with success in curing people with lead poisoning who were working in battery plants, and the U.S. Navy used it on people who had acquired lead poisoning from repainting old ships. Not only did EDTA eliminate the poisoning, but physicians noted that patients also showed considerable improvement in cardiovascular symptoms. The FDA has approved EDTA for the treatment of lead poisoning, hypercalcemia, and heart attacks caused by digitalis poisoning. EDTA is legally available for a physician's use and it is quite legal for a licensed physician to utilize a drug for any purpose, which, in that physician's judgment, is best for the patient. Thus, since the 1960s, EDTA has been used to treat cardiovascular disease coupled with dietary changes and nutritional supplements.

Only licensed physicians are able to provide chelation therapy in the United States. In some facilities the physicians oversee the procedure, which is actually implemented by registered nurses. The American Heart Association does not approve of chelation therapy. The conventional approach to treating severe atherosclerosis is angioplasty, a mechanical method of scrubbing the inside of clogged arteries with an inflated balloon catheter to flatten the deposits of plaque, or bypass surgery.

In early experiments, EDTA was often used in doses up to 10 times the amount now recommended. This resulted in serious adverse effects, including renal failure. With the lower doses and with the use of kidney function tests, and by following recommended protocols, the present-day procedure is considered to be safe.

Chelation therapy is performed in an outpatient or physician's office setting. EDTA is given as an intravenous infusion over a period of 3–4 hours. Usually 20– treatments, at an average cost of $80 to $100 each, are administered at the rate of 1–3 sessions per week. The average cost of a course of treatment is $3,000 to $5,000, compared to the average cost of balloon angioplasty at $12,000 and bypass surgery in excess of $30,000.

In late 1996, an oral chelation substance was introduced to the market. It is a three-month program designed to detoxify and balance the cardiovascular system. The oral route is advisable for people with potential heart problems but whose condition does not yet require rapid action. The advantages of oral chelation are that it does not require a physician's supervision or expensive blood tests to monitor and is much lower in cost. The primary disadvantage is the longer time to get the same benefits as intravenous chelation.

Getting Started with Purification Therapies

Sweating, as a natural method of purification, can be helpful for many people, especially those who smoke, drink, or use other drugs, suffer chemical exposures, or eat a lot of salt. The complete recommended program is to exercise for 20 minutes, sauna or steam bath for a maximum of 30 minutes, take a cleansing shower, and then have a massage. Be careful as you emerge from the sauna or steam bath as you may be weak, dizzy, or unstable on your feet. It is especially important that you drink plenty of water throughout the program to replace the fluids that are lost. Even after the sweat, fluid intake should be high, to continue the flushing out of toxins and to prevent dehydration.

Steam inhalation is an excellent remedy for respiratory problems such as chest congestion, bronchitis, bronchial cough, laryngitis, and sinusitis. Adding sage and eucalyptus to the steam is both soothing and antibacterial, which decreases the chance of secondary bacterial infection in viral respiratory diseases. Steam inhalation can be done with a commercial steam vaporizer or through making one's own steam tent. A towel draped over one's head and over the top of a pot of boiling water is quite effective. Great care must be taken not to set the towel on fire if the source of heat is a gas burner.

Hot, wet compresses are good treatment for localized infections. Simply wet a towel, wring it out, and heat it in the microwave. Care must be taken to avoid temperatures hot enough to burn. Place on the infected area for 15 minutes at least three or four times a day. Heat is also effective for sore muscles as well as menstrual and intestinal cramps. This therapy can be accomplished with heating pads or with gel packs designed to be heated in a microwave. Cold compresses are good for bruises, sprains, traumatized joints, burns, bites, and stings. A package of frozen peas wrapped in a towel makes a excellent cold compress. A home first aid kit should include a gel ice pack that can be stored in the freezer until it is needed. For campers, instant ice packs are available and simply need to be squeezed, stretched, and applied. A cold compress will reduce leakage of fluid into injured tissues, reduce swelling and pain, and slow the spread of any toxins into the system. It should be kept in place for most of the first few hours and then used intermittently for 24 hours after the injury.

Intense sweating at the very start of a viral infection may greatly reduce the severity of the illness. A sauna or steam bath produces the most effective sweating, but you can approximate that kind of therapy at home. Try prewarming your bed with an electric blanket or other means, and then fill the bathtub with comfortably hot water between 102 and 104 degrees Fahrenheit. Submerge your body as much as possible for 15 minutes, then towel off and jump into the prewarmed bed, covering up to stay warm, and resting for at least one hour. This sequence can be done as often as two or three times a day to treat a cold or the flu.

Colonic and chelation therapies are not suitable for home experimentation and should be administered only by a professional. See the resources section for more information.

TRY IT YOURSELF: DETOXIFYING BATHS

A number of substances can be added to the bath to help detoxify the body. The sulfur component of Epsom salts helps to rid the body of toxins as well as to increase sweating and increase the blood supply to the skin's surface. Begin with one-fourth cup of Epsom salts per bath and gradually increase until you are using 4 cups per bath. Apple-cider vinegar changes the pH of the skin, which aids in the detoxification process. Again, it is best to begin with one-fourth cup and gradually increase to one cup. Baking soda baths, one cup per bath, are alkalinizing and good for cleansing and drying weeping, open sores.

Ginger root baths increase sweating and help draw toxins to the skin surface. Cut a thumb size piece of ginger root in small pieces. These pieces should be put in a pot of water and brought to a boil. Turn off the heat and steep for 30 minutes. Strain the solution and pour into the bath. Any number of herbs can be brewed as a cup of tea and then added to the bath, which should only include one herb at a time. The most popular herbal baths are catnip, yarrow, peppermint, boneset, blessed thistle, pleurisy root, chamomile, blue vervain, and horsetail. Once your detoxifying ingredient is prepared, use the following procedure to make the most of it. Always make sure that someone else is in the house, since lightheadedness and dizziness can result from hot baths.

- Wash the body thoroughly in a shower before the bath; rinse thoroughly.
- Have the bath water as hot as tolerable without burning, 102–104°F. Add your detoxifying formula once the bath is drawn.
- Begin with a 5-minute soak; gradually build up the time over a number of baths until you can soak for 30 minutes.
- Drink 8 ounces of water during the bath.
- After soaking, take a cleansing shower; scrub with soap and rinse well to remove the toxins that have been excreted on the skin.
- Follow this procedure three times a week until your health has improved, and then one or two times a week to reduce stress and maintain health.

THE ABSOLUTE MINIMUM

- Most physicians agree: There's nothing like a nice hot (or cold) bath. By promoting sweating to draw out toxins from the skin, altering the flow of blood through the body, and easing breathing, bathing can not only remove health-threatening agents, but also promote a deeper feeling of relaxation and well-being.

- Proponents of colon hydrotherapy argue that flushing material from the large intestine reduces the stress that digestion and environmental toxins put on the body. Colonic cleansing should always be performed by a professional.

- Chelation therapy uses a synthetic amino acid, EDTA, to binds to and remove heavy metals from the bloodstream. Its proponents, including the physicians who must administer the treatments, believe that it detoxifies and balances the cardiovascular system

RESOURCES

- American Board of Chelation Therapy

  www.abct.info

- American College for Advancement in Medicine

  www.acam.org

- International Association for Colon Hydrotherapy

  www.i-act.org

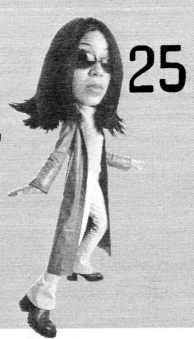

25

Animal-Assisted Therapy

Animal-Assisted Therapy (AAT) is defined as the use of specifically selected animals as a treatment method in health and human service settings. AAT has been steadily gaining in popularity in the United States and has been shown to be a successful intervention for people with a variety of physical or psychological conditions. Despite reluctance and skepticism on the part of many administrators of health care facilities, nurses have often advocated the use of animals as a therapeutic intervention. One of the earliest recorded observations of a connection between animals and health was made by Florence Nightingale in 1860 when she noted, "a small pet is often an excellent companion for the sick, for long chronic cases especially." She further suggested that whenever possible, patients should participate in the care of the animal because this activity was helpful to their recovery. Long banned from health care facilities, dogs, cats, and other pets are gradually being welcomed with open arms.

What Is Animal-Assisted Therapy?

The York Retreat in England, founded in 1792 for the treatment of people with mental illness, used small animals such as rabbits and poultry in their treatment plan. The goal was to decrease the use of restraints and medications by helping residents learn self-control through animals that relied on them for care. Bethel, a residential treatment center for people with epilepsy, founded in 1867 in Germany, utilized pets as an important part of the treatment program. This pet program is still in place today and has expanded to include farm animals and a wild game park. In the United States in the 1940s, injured World War II soldiers were encouraged to work with the hogs, cattle, and horses on the farm of the Army Air Corps Convalescent Hospital in New York. Since that time, animals have been used in many U.S. clinical settings from pediatrics to geriatrics, acute-care facilities to chronic care homes, from group accommodations to private homes, from prevention to healing, and even from schools to correctional facilities nationwide.

note

In the 1990s, the Delta Society developed the first comprehensive standards of practice for animal-assisted therapy. Now in its second edition, *Standards of Practice for Animal-Assisted Activities and Animal-Assisted Therapy* defines the role of animals in therapeutic programs.

What Kinds of Animals Are Used?

Therapy dogs and cats are specifically selected for temperament, companionability, and interaction. Temperament is the animal's natural or instinctive behavior and is important in terms of the way the animal will react when stressed. A good therapy pet is calm, tolerant, and friendly. The second major criterion is that the animal has a person who is willing to volunteer time and energy in order to share the pet with others. Dogs must be trained in obedience prior to participating in the program. A dog or cat must be at least one year of age before enrolling in the training and visiting program to better ensure that the pet has been effectively socialized and is comfortable interacting with numerous people in a crowded setting. In addition, the animal's immune system is more stabilized by this age.

A veterinarian must verify the animal's health and inoculations must be current. AAT-registering organizations require that a dog and its handler pass several tests prior to registration. In general, dogs have to demonstrate basic obedience skills and must be indifferent to crowds and distractions and unfazed by exuberant or clumsy handling, including ear tugging and "bear hugging." In addition, they must have a high tolerance for unfamiliar or loud noises and peculiar smells. Therapeutic riding horses must have a gentle, tolerant temperament, be well balanced and well muscled, and move with even strides. In addition to the familiar dogs and cats in pet therapy, other animals may include parrots, cockatoos, guinea pigs, rabbits, potbellied pigs, dwarf goats, llamas, donkeys, and horses.

Animal handler volunteers are trained in workshops or through home study courses. The handlers must pass a written test and their animals must pass a skills test. Participation in continuing education is required. Nurses, physical and occupational therapists, psychotherapists, and other health care professionals must receive training to direct animal-assisted therapy programs. This educational process is still in the beginning stages, and at this time is primarily accomplished through in-service training, and seminars and workshops at national and international professional meetings.

Twelve countries, including the United States, offer formalized educational programs for registration, certification, or licensure of therapists. These programs have intermittent sessions, which may span one to two years. Most frequently this specialized training is offered to physical therapists, occupational therapists, psychotherapists, and special education teachers.

What's the Idea Behind Animal-Assisted Therapy?

The characteristics that make many pets cherished family members—unconditional affection, responsiveness, and companionability—also make pets effective in therapy. Animal-assisted therapy brings pets into a healing context in a way that's safe and effective for both patient and pet.

Companion Animals: Part of the Family

Many people think of their animals as surrogate children, with one big exception: These are children who rarely, if ever, disappoint their parents. Pets, especially dogs, often seem to understand what their owners are feeling. For some people, a pet is a reason to get up in the morning. It is something to nurture, touch, and stroke. For stress relief, it apparently does not matter much whether the pet is a Labrador, a cat, or a canary. What is most important is the person's relationship with the pet.

The contributions companion animals make to the emotional well-being of people include providing unconditional love and opportunities for affection; functioning as a confidant, playmate, and companion; and assisting in the achievement of trust, responsibility, and empathy toward others. Studies of children with pets indicate that the unconditional love and acceptance conveyed in the child-animal relationship may validate a child's sense of self-worth. In addition, older school-age children often turn to companion animals in times of stress for reassurance. Children often perceive their companion animals as play partners, most often during middle childhood than during adolescence or early childhood.

Children with interactive pets such as dogs and cats are more attached to their companion animals than are children with other types of pets such as hamsters, fish, and turtles. Emotional bonds are more likely to be formed with animals that are able to respond in an outwardly loving and affectionate way. Behaviors like tail wagging, barking, and purring often bring out affectionate responses in human caregivers. In North America and Europe, pets are found in the majority of homes with children. Families with children, especially school-age children, are more likely to own companion animals than are families without children. Multiple-pet ownership is also common. Pet ownership remains higher in rural versus urban areas, and in houses versus apartments. Still, across a variety of settings, the majority of children in Western countries are living with companion animals.

Therapy Animals: Part of the Healing Process

In this age of high technological health care, it is sometimes easy to forget the importance of unconditional affection. Animals pay little attention to age or physical ability, but accept people as they are. It is insignificant if the person has no hair, is in a wheelchair, or is hallucinating. The underlying concept that supports the use of animals for therapeutic reasons is the bonding experience it provides. Frail or depressed older adults often brighten up and adopt a more positive outlook when they are in the presence of an animal "therapist."

Many health care professionals are finding that loneliness may be as serious as cancer and heart disease for older adults. Older people who stay active, find substitutes for work, and build new relationships as partners and friends die have been found most satisfied with life. Not all older adults, however, have options for remaining active and forming new friendships. Visiting with animals can help people feel less lonely and less depressed. Animals can provide a welcome change from routine or a distraction from disability or pain. People often talk to the animals and share with them their thoughts, feelings, and memories. When people talk to people, their blood pressure tends to go up because of questions of how one is being evaluated or judged. With animals, who are always eager to please, and unconditionally accepting, a person's blood pressure tends to go down.

Animals also make it easier for two strangers to talk. They give people a common interest, provide a focus for conversation, and broaden the circle of friends. Residents laugh and mingle more when animals visit long-term care facilities than when the animals are not there. Animals also help stimulate socialization by providing an opportunity to share stories of animals the residents may have had in the past. Many people like to stroke the animal while talking about the pets that shared their lives.

Three significant problems that manifest within traditional long-term care facilities are loneliness, helplessness, and boredom. They often have not served as homes for people, but rather as institutions in which to store them. Residents may be intensely lonely, with long stretches of empty time. The basic concept of the Eden Alternative—a new approach to long-term care—is quite simple: Long-term care facilities are viewed as habitats for human beings rather than institutions for the frail and elderly. The Eden Alternative seeks to eliminate the problems of loneliness, helplessness, and boredom by providing interaction with companion animals, the opportunity to care for other living things, and a milieu of variety and spontaneity. "Edenized" facilities share a commitment to change the system, and not just through "fur and feathers." Quality of life is emphasized as much as the quality of care. Residents and employees alike are encouraged to play a role in making that quality atmosphere happen. Administrators recognize that the care a resident receives is usually completed in three to four hours of the day, leaving 20 hours to live a life. As the U.S. population ages, and with growing frustration with traditional systems, long-term care facilities will have to be managed far differently than they are today. The Eden Alternative is the most innovative reform effort to date.

What Are the Goals of Animal-Assisted Therapy?

In AAT, an accredited professional guides the human-animal interaction toward specific, individualized therapeutic goals. In one treatment session, a variety of goals can be addressed: physical goals such as range of motion, balance, and mobility; cognitive goals such as improved memory or verbal expression; emotional goals such as increased self-esteem and motivation; and social goals such as building rapport and improved socialization skills. Linda Hume, L.P.N., an AAT specialist, has developed a program of animal facilitation in occupational and physical therapy at Northeast Rehabilitation Hospital in Salem, New Hampshire. The following are a few of the goals and activities she has identified for AAT in her clinical setting:

- Increased upper extremity range of motion: Throw an object for dog to retrieve; use of leash to maneuver dog; pet, stroke, brush animal

- Mobility: Ambulate with dog

- Improved coordination: Throw an object for dog to retrieve (releasing); reaching for object dog has retrieved

- Improved memory: Asked to recall dog's name, breed, age, etc.; commanding dog to sit and remembering to release dog from command

- Increased language production: Use of commands with dog; simply conversing to or about animal
- Object identification: Direct dog to retrieve specific familiar items by appropriate name—ball, spoon, pen, or cup, for example
- Attention/Concentration: Attending to dog, task, and therapist

Therapeutic horseback riding, available in at least 21 countries, is defined as rehabilitative use of horses. In equine-assisted psychotherapy, the riding is designed to support the psychotherapeutic treatment plan. Goals include increased self-confidence, improved self-esteem, refined social competence, the experience of pleasure, and the ability to establish a relationship with the horse. Remedial educational riding is used to further the educational and behavioral goals for school-age children with learning problems. The horse is used as a strong motivator for accomplishing specific treatment goals. Hippotherapy is the use of the rhythmic movement of the horse to increase sensory processing and improve posture, balance, and mobility in people with movement dysfunctions. The term derives from the Greek word "hippo" meaning horse. The transfer of movement from the horse to the client is designed primarily to achieve physical goals but may also affect psychological, cognitive, behavioral, and communication outcomes. Clients benefiting from hippotherapy include adults and children with cerebral palsy, multiple sclerosis, orthopedic problems, posttraumatic spasticity, strokes, scoliosis, genetic syndromes, and developmental delays, among others.

Animal-Assisted Activities

A less formal approach, known as Animal-Assisted Activities (AAA), is motivational, educational, and recreational. The goal is to provide "meeting and greeting" human-animal interactions to enhance the quality of life, rather than a specific treatment plan. AAA is used in many types of facilities with a wide variety of animals. AAA visits to sheltered homeless families have been effective. Most shelters do not allow families to bring their pets, and seeing the visiting animal can be therapeutic, especially for children. AAA visits give homeless children a chance to participate in everyday experiences they may not have had recently, like walking a dog or playing fetch.

Pet Visits

A family pet visit is the arrangement for a pet to visit the owner in the health care setting. The concept of a pet visit as therapy for hospitalized people is not new, especially in facilities with rehabilitation and mental health units. The pet that visits may belong to a pet therapy program or may be the client's own pet. The University of Utah Hospital in Salt Lake City has had a pet visitation policy for many years. They believe that allowing a pet to visit can be a healing experience for patients, family members, and even the pet. Pets are even allowed to visit in ICU settings, with the approval of the nurses, and if the patient's medical condition doesn't prevent the visit.

Resident Animals

A resident animal lives at the health care facility. The staff is responsible for the complete health and well-being of the animal and residents are included in providing routine daily care. Grooming and brushing, for example, are good therapies for the hands. Some staff reports that full-time pets become so perceptive that they actually gravitate to the rooms of people who are the most isolated or depressed. Those residents who have regular visits are more receptive to treatment, have a greater incentive to recover, and have an increased will to live.

Eden Alternative

In the Eden Alternative, nursing homes are places where the residents give as well as receive care and where a diversity of species create a natural habitat. The approach uses animals, plants, and children to interact with residents of long-term care centers, creating a "human habitat" that makes the residents feel more at home—and not so much in one. Resident animals are part of the total environment. Children and teenagers from schools and youth volunteer programs frequently visit the home. They come in and interact and build relationships with residents, as opposed to the usual pattern of coming in, putting on a program, and leaving.

The Eden Alternative empowers residents and the staff members who come into daily contact with them. Residents have more say in their activities, menus, and daily routines; caregivers, maintenance workers, and other employees can set their own work schedules, within given parameters. Supporters of the program believe that employees frequently seem happier in Eden homes as evidenced by fewer sick days and lower staff turnover. The Eden Alternative is really about liberating the spirit of the people who are living and working in long-term care.

The movement remains loosely organized, spreading largely by word of mouth. North Carolina has declared unofficially that it is an Eden Alternative state and has assembled a special coalition giving financial aid grants to encourage facilities to adopt Eden techniques. The Lt. Governor of Missouri, Roger B. Wilson, has asked the state's Division of Aging to help promote Eden. About 60 facilities there are in the process of implementing programs. Eden programs are also popular in New York, where William Thomas, M.D., founded the approach. Eden Alternative got its start in nursing homes but has grown to include adult day care services and assisted-living facilities (Levine, 1997).

Service Dogs

Service dogs are individually trained to do work or perform tasks for a person with a physical or emotional disability. They legally may go anywhere that a person with disabilities goes. Most people are familiar with guide dogs for those with visual impairment. Other service dogs can be trained to pull a wheelchair, open doors, retrieve dropped objects as small as a dime, and turn light switches on and off. Hearing dogs alert owners to important sounds that need a response. Seizure response dogs recognize behaviors associated with their owner's seizures and can be trained to stay with the person or get help. When breathing machines malfunction, service dogs can be trained to nose the phone receiver out of its cradle and hit the speed-dial buttons, all of which are programmed to 911. Training service dogs is an expensive and time-consuming project. The dog spends the first year of life with a foster family who is responsible for socialization and basic obedience training. Next comes five to six months of intensive training followed by six months of in-home training with the new owner. The benefit, of course, is that people can lead more independent and fulfilling lives.

In correctional institutes all across Ohio, puppies and prisoners are teaming up in an unusual program. A nonprofit organization called Pilot Dogs, Inc., places service puppies under the care of prisoners until the pups are ready for formal training as service dogs. Since the inception of the program in 1992, some 250 dogs have been placed in prisons. Inmates are chosen based on their records of good behavior and experience with dogs. No violent offenders are permitted to raise the dogs. The puppies sleep in crates in the cells with their partners and accompany them on their daily activities, including trips to the dining hall where the puppies learn to be well behaved around people and become accustomed to the noise and crowds they will face later. The prisoner is responsible for the care and well-being of the dog, housebreaking them, leash-training them, and putting them through a basic obedience course. After spending about 12 months at the correctional facility, the puppies are removed and placed in an intensive training program. A major advantage for the dogs is having human contact 24 hours a day, which is less likely to occur in regular foster homes. The chosen prisoners have the pleasure and delight of having a puppy to give love to and get love from. They also have the satisfaction of seeing the benefits of their training as the puppies progress.

Special Concerns for Pet Owners with HIV/AIDS

In the past, individuals with HIV and/or AIDS have been told to give up their pets for fear that their compromised immune system would place them at high risk for zoonotic infections. The reality is that people are more likely to contract zoonotic infections from contaminated food, water, soil, or even other people than from pets. The HIV virus only infects humans and other primates and, therefore, cannot be spread from or to dogs, cats, birds, or even fish.

With proper care and understanding and a healthy pet, the potential health risks of pet companionship are minimal and the benefits may far outweigh the risks. People living with HIV often deal with feelings of isolation, rejection, and lack of purpose. For such people, companion animals offer purpose, a feeling of being needed, a way to increase socialization, and a constant source of unconditional affection. When selecting a pet, consider a pet with the temperament, energy level, and environmental needs that matches your own. An older pet may be more appropriate than a young one. You also need to follow some simple guidelines when caring for your pet and yourself. The precautions are designed to protect an immunocompromised person from acquiring secondary infections.

Veterinary Care

- Have your veterinarian examine your pet initially, and then at least once a year.
- Keep your pet up to date on annual shots and rabies vaccination.
- Seek veterinary care immediately for sick pets.
- Street animals that you "adopt" should be checked by a veterinarian before bringing them into your home.

Pet Care

- Keep your pet clean and well groomed with short, blunt toenails.
- Keep the pet's living and feeding areas clean.
- Keep your cat's litter box out of the kitchen; use a litter box liner and change it daily.
- Always walk your pet on a leash and minimize the pet's contact with other animals and garbage.
- Cats should be kept indoors and be prevented from hunting birds and rodents.

- Feed your pet only commercially prepared pet foods; never feed raw meat or unpasteurized milk.

- Do not allow birds to fly free in your home; you must avoid their droppings.

General Hygiene

- Wash your hands frequently, especially before eating, smoking, or attending to open wounds.

- Keep your cat off all kitchen surfaces. If not possible, be sure to wipe down, with a gentle disinfectant, any surface where you may place your food.

- Do not allow your dog to drink out of the toilet because it is a place of many germs.

- Try to avoid contact with your pet's bodily fluids. Gloves and a breathing mask should be worn for clean up including cleaning a litter box, aquarium, or bird cage.

INTERACTING WITH YOUR PET

When you are feeling tense or anxious and if you have a dog or a cat to whom you are attached, try this:

- Note your physical and emotional signs of tension: Are your hands clenched? Is your body trembling? Are you restlessness? Are you unable to relax? Do you have a mouth dry, stomach upset, or breathing rapidly? Are you unable to concentrate? Are your worrying? You can also have a friend take your pulse and blood pressure.

- Do something with your pet for at least 20 minutes, for example, play, groom, or talk.

- Have your friend take your pulse and blood pressure again and compare the results to those taken prior to the interaction. Then conduct another self-assessment. What, if anything, has changed?

THE ABSOLUTE MINIMUM

- The unconditional love and affection demonstrated by pets has a profoundly positive impact on physical and psychological healing.

- Animal-assisted therapies bring these benefits to patients, pets, and pet owners in a variety of contexts, including hospitals, rehabilitation facilities, hospices, and the homes of long term patients such as those with HIV/AIDS.

RESOURCES

- American Hippotherapy Association

  www.americanequestrian.com/hippotherapy.htm

- The Delta Society

  www.deltasociety.org

- Pet Owners with HIV/AIDS Resource Service, Inc. (POWARS)

  www.thebody.com/powars/powars.html

PART VIII

APPENDIX

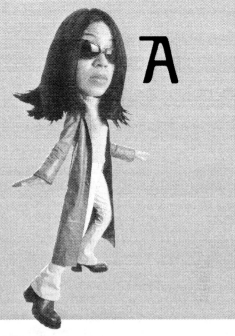

ALTERNATIVE THERAPIES FOR COMMON HEALTH PROBLEMS

These types of problems often respond well to alternative therapies and lifestyle modification. If in doubt of the seriousness of symptoms, see your health care practitioner. A number of suggestions are given for various problems. Select one that seems to be the most appropriate for your situation and keep notes on what seems to work and what does not. Modify these suggestions according to your individual needs.

Abrasions, Scrapes

▓ Aromatherapy: after washing with soap and water, apply 1–3 drops of lavender or tea tree oil to wound; reapply 2 times a day until healed

▓ To disinfect, pour 3% hydrogen peroxide into the wound and let it foam up

▓ Apply the skin of a freshly peeled banana to the affected area, or cut a thin slice of raw potato and tape it over the affected area

▓ Herbs: sprinkle goldenseal powder in wound, crushed garlic mixed with honey makes a soothing salve—spread on a piece of clean gauze and cover the injured area

Acne

▓ Aromatherapy: bergamot, cedarwood, chamomile, clary sage, lemon grass, melissa, patchouli, rosemary, sandalwood, tea tree, thyme, ylang-ylang—can be made into a facial mask, compress, or topical cream; tea tree oil and lavender can be applied directly to blemishes

▓ Herbs: arnica, calendula skin products

▓ Drink plenty of water to flush out the system

▓ Supplements: 500 units of vitamin A, 5 mg zinc, or 1500 mg evening primrose oil

AIDS

▓ Acupuncture

▓ Herbs: curcumin, extract of boxwood plant

▓ Massage

▓ Supplements: Iron, vitamins C, E, and Bs; beta carotene, glutamine, selenium

Allergies

▓ Applied Kinesiology

▓ Herbs: stinging nettles to lessen runny nose and sneezing; teas made from chamomile, elder, or yarrow flowers can reduce reactions

▓ Homeopathy: allium cepa (onion); windflower, for swelling in the face—1 tablet of apis every 15 minutes—maximum 6 doses

▓ Supplements: vitamin C to decrease histamine production

Alzheimer's Disease (Dementia)

- Herbs: ginkgo 120–240 mg daily
- Supplements: zinc, selenium, evening primrose oil

Alcohol Abuse

- Acupuncture
- Herbs: milk thistle, kudzu
- Meditation
- Yoga

Amputations: Phantom Pain

- Magnets: improve blood flow to stump and cause phantom pain to disappear
- Massage

Anxiety

- Acupressure: press center of inside wrist 1 inch above crease toward elbow
- Animal-assisted therapy
- Aromatherapy: basil, bergamot, chamomile, frankincense deepens breathing to induce calmness, green apple, juniper, lemon balm, orange, neroli for panic attacks
- Biofeedback
- Healing Touch
- Herbs: valerian, passion flower, kava kava
- Homeopathy: St. Ignatius bean, arsenic
- Massage
- Meditation
- Reiki
- Relaxation techniques
- Therapeutic Touch
- Performance anxiety—hypnosis, guided imagery, Alexander Technique

Arthritis

- Aromatherapy: cedarwood, coriander, cypress massage or cold compress, compress of rosemary to swollen joints
- Exercise in water (nonweight-bearing) or moderate exercise as tolerated
- Feldenkrais Method
- Herbs: devil's claw, boswellia, evening primrose oil; ginger; capsaicin cream applied topically, glucosamine (1500 mg) and chondroitin (1200 mg) to help restore joint integrity; natural anti-inflammatories like willowbark, turmeric, and ginger
- Homeopathy: poison ivy
- Ice joints and then rub in analgesic oils
- Magnets placed over an inflamed area on regular basis
- Reflexology: all joints of the hands and feet should be worked for pain relief and mobility of corresponding body joints
- Supplements: thiamine; vitamins B6, B12
- Therapeutic Touch
- Yoga: practice slowly, seeing how far the affected joints can be moved without pain; do not exercise joints when they are inflamed

Asthma

- Acupuncture
- Alexander Technique: teaches a more relaxed way of breathing and enables you to manage yourself better during an asthma attack
- Aromatherapy: put several drops of cypress on a handkerchief and inhale deeply; put frankincense on a pillow at night to slow and deepen the breathing
- Biofeedback
- Breathing exercises
- Hypnosis
- Herbs: holy basil, elecampine, country mallow, malabar nut, bayberry; mix 3 parts tincture of lobelia with 1 part tincture of capsicum—take 20 drops in water at the start of an asthmatic attack—repeat every 30 minutes for a total of 3 or 4 doses

■ Homeopathy: Arsenicum album, 1 tablet 3 times daily; maximum 1 week

■ Meditation

■ Reflexology: during an asthma attack, work the reflexes for the diaphragm and lungs on the balls of the feet

■ Water: drink plenty of water to keep the respiratory tract secretions fluid

■ Yoga: focus on expansive postures and breathing practices designed to increase the length of the exhalation

Athlete's Foot

■ Acupressure: do full foot or hand acupressure massage session twice a week to stimulate the immune and endocrine systems; do not press on broken, sore, or cracked skin areas

■ Aromatherapy: cedarwood, lemon balm, rosemary; mix 2 drops lavender oil and 1 drop tea tree oil and apply between toes

■ Herbs: black walnut tincture—apply directly to fungus patches and drink a tea of green crushed walnut hulls for fungus anywhere in body

■ Naturopathy: take 2 Kyolic garlic tablets TID, decrease to BID when all infections are healed; dust your feet and shoes with garlic powder

■ Supplements: take B-complex vitamins, 50–100 TID with meals; dust vitamin C powder directly onto affected area; zinc may help clear the skin and boost the immune system

Attention Deficit Disorder

■ Biofeedback

■ Supplements: B vitamins

Back Pain

■ Acupuncture

■ Alexander Technique: teaches a more balanced used of body since muscular imbalance often contributes to back pain

■ Applied kinesiology

■ Biofeedback

- Chiropractic manipulation
- Herbs: valerian, nutmeg, gotu kola; to ease local discomfort soak a compress in 1/2 cup hot water containing 1 tbsp. camp bark and 1 tsp. cinnamon tinctures
- Homeopathy: 4 tablets of arnica as soon as possible after an injury and repeat every hour for the first day while awake, second day—4 tablets every 2 hours; third day—4 tablets four times
- Hydrotherapy: for acute back pain, use an ice pack on affected area for 20 minutes every 1–2 hours
- Magnets: place small magnets over area of muscle spasm in back
- Massage with warm oil
- Reflexology: work the spinal reflexes, especially the tender points, on the medial longitudinal arches of the feet (the bony ridges on the inside)
- Sleep on back with pillows under knees or on side with pillow between bent knees
- Yoga: lie down with legs bent, feet flat on floor, exhale fully and slowly for at least 12 breaths; long-term yoga practice can strengthen back muscles

Balance Problems

- Qigong
- T'ai Chi
- Hippotherapy

Bee Stings/Insect Bites

- Aromatherapy: tea tree, basil, bergamot, lavender, thyme, ylang-ylang
- Add enough water to baking soda or meat tenderizer to make a paste and apply it to the sting
- Cover affected area with a small amount of mashed fresh papaya
- Herbs: apply fresh aloe vera sap directly to the bite; if bite becomes infected, bathe with marigold or echinacea tea; apply a fresh slice of onion to both bee and wasp stings; a mixture of honey and crushed garlic makes a soothing ointment
- Homeopathy: Apis, 1 tablet every 30 minutes, maximum 6 doses for burning and swelling

Bones (Broken)

- Aromatherapy: massage in elemi oil prior to casting
- Bioelectromagnetics: place magnets into the dressings over fractures
- Healing Touch
- Reiki
- Therapeutic Touch

Bruises

- Aromatherapy: cypress, combine 1 drop of chamomile with 2 tsp. of ice cold water—soak a cotton pad and apply to affected area
- Herbs: witch hazel (topical), arnica tablets or massage tincture of arnica into bruised area; 200–400 mg three times a day of bromelain on an empty stomach
- Homeopathy: aconite, 1 or 2 doses only over 15 minutes immediately for the "shock" of the injury
- Hydrotherapy: cold compresses for first 12 hours with occasional breaks to prevent excessive chilling
- Supplements: 2,000 mg vitamin C three times a day for people who bruise easily; pineapple juice—enzymes speed the rate at which the blood causing the bruise dissolves

Burns (Minor)

- Aromatherapy: for pain relief—chamomile, eucalyptus, geranium, lavender; to reduce inflammation—chamomile, clary sage, geranium, lavender, myrrh, tea tree; to regenerate skin—chamomile, clary sage, eucalyptus, geranium, myrrh, rose, tea tree
- Herbs: aloe vera sap, calendula lotion, or raw honey
- Hydrotherapy: immediately immerse the affected part in ice water for 5–10 minutes with brief break during the first 20 minutes after the injury
- Magnets: place over site of injury to control pain and speed healing

Cancer

■ Antioxidants: vitamins A, C, and E; Co-enzyme 10

■ Imagery

■ Massage

■ Meditation

■ Qigong

■ Yoga

Canker Sores

■ Herbs: mix 1 cup of warm water with 1/4 teaspoon of salt and 1/2 teaspoon of goldenseal powder; licorice root gel, echinacea tincture, butternut, comfrey

■ Supplements: vitamin A (25,000–50,000 IU daily) prevents infection from spreading; B-complex (50–100 IU TID); vitamin E (400–800 IU daily); selenium (200 mcg daily); acidophilus, 4 capsules, 4–6 times per day

Carpal Tunnel Syndrome

■ Chiropractic manipulation

■ Herbs: ginger compress

■ Magnets placed over the front and back of the wrist to control symptoms

■ Massage

■ Pressure-point therapies

Chest Congestion

■ Aromatherapy: cedarwood, steam inhalation of eucalyptus, frankincense; massage chest with lavender, inhale marjoram, peppermint, eucalyptus, or rosemary, drops of tea tree on handkerchief

■ Herbs: tea made with peppermint and yarrow (1/2 tsp. each); sage or eucalyptus leaves in a bowl of steaming water—inhale with a towel draped over the head

■ Magnets: wear on chest over bronchial tubes and at equal level on the back; sleeping on a magnetic mattress pad can be helpful

Cholesterol (High)

- Herbs: garlic, Indian gooseberry
- Meditation
- Supplements: Profibe (grapefruit fiber)
- Yoga

Circulation (Poor)

- Aromatherapy: rosemary (increases circulation to skin), vetiver
- Biofeedback
- Exercise
- Healing Touch
- Herbs: ginkgo, garlic, cayenne, hawthorn, bilberry
- Hypnosis
- Imagery
- Magnets
- Massage
- Therapeutic Touch
- Yoga

Common Cold

- Acupressure: if sinuses become blocked or painful
- Aromatherapy: inhale lavender, eucalyptus, or peppermint oil in steam vaporizer to speed recovery and lessens stuffiness; add 3 drops lemon oil, 2 drops thyme and tea tree oil, and 1 drop eucalyptus into hot bath
- Herbs: tea from fresh ginger and brown sugar, echinacea at the first sign of a cold, astragalus, garlic, goldenseal
- Homeopathy: allium cepa (onion), monkshood, aconite, or natrum muriaticum: 1 tablet up to every 4 hours, as needed—maximum 3–4 days.
- Reflexology: work the fingers and thumbs, the webs between the fingers, the pads beneath the fingers, and the spaces on the back of the hands for the reflexes of the head, lungs, and upper lymphatics
- Supplements: vitamin C, zinc lozenges

Cold Sores

- Aromatherapy: apply tea tree oil at onset and continue until cleared
- Herbs: lemon-balm tea shows significant antiviral activity against herpes simplex; echinacea (600 mg daily) or goldenseal (100 mg daily)

Colic

- Aromatherapy: chamomile (rubbed on abdomen), coriander, orange, peppermint
- Massage abdomen; massage bottom of feet with warmed sesame oil

Constipation

- Aromatherapy: massage abdomen in a clockwise direction with orange, black pepper, ginger, or marjoram mixed in a carrier oil
- Exercise: especially activities that work the abdominal muscles such as rowing, swimming, walking, or sit-ups
- Herbs: dandelion root, chicory root, angelica root (20–30 drops of extract in a small glass of water three times a day), cascara sagrada, senna; psyllium—only use for several days, long-term use can be damaging
- Homeopathy: bryonia (wild hops) or nux vomica—1 tablet 3 times daily—maximum 1 week
- Drink 6–8 glasses of water daily
- Yoga: twisting postures and forward bends are often helpful

Corns

- Aromatherapy: mix 2 drops each of orange, lemon, and lavender oils in a basin of warm water and soak feet for at least 15 minutes per day

Cough

- Aromatherapy: cedarwood; several drops of cypress or tea tree on handkerchief and inhale deeply; add 3 drops eucalyptus and 2 drops thyme oil to 2 tsp. vegetable oil—massage into neck and chest; steam inhalation using sandalwood, benzoin, eucalyptus, or frankincense

- Herbs: licorice, wild cherry bark, thyme; tincture of mullein in warm water three times a day
- Homeopathy: bryonia (wild hops), monkshood, rumex, stannum—1 tablet 3 times daily until improved—maximum 2 weeks
- Reflexology: work the lung and diaphragm reflexes on and beneath balls of feet and webs between big toes and second toes

Depression

- Acupuncture
- Animal-assisted therapy
- Aromatherapy: bergamot, geranium, jasmine, lemon balm, rose, ylang-ylang; to bath add 15 drops geranium, 10 drops of bergamot, and 5 drops of lavender
- Exercise
- Flower essences: gentian, hornbeam, mustard, gorse, sweet chestnut
- Healing Touch
- Herbs: St. John's wort, valerian
- Meditation
- Reiki
- Supplements: B vitamins
- T'ai Chi
- Therapeutic Touch
- Transcranial magnetic stimulation

Diabetes

- Biofeedback
- Exercise
- Herbs: blueberry leaf tea, 2 cups a day on a regular basis; 100–200 mg of co-enzyme Q every day for a least 3 months to stabilize blood sugar
- Yoga

Diarrhea

- Aromatherapy: coriander, chamomile, neroli, lavender, or peppermint in carrier oil—gentle abdominal massage
- Herbs: 2 tsp. per cup of boiling water to make tea of black pepper, chamomile, coriander, rosemary, sandalwood, or thyme
- Homeopathy: podophyllum—1 tablet hourly until improved, then every 4 hours—maximum 5 days
- Supplements: zinc
- Replace lost fluids

Ear Infections

- Acupressure: massage just behind the tip of the mastoid bone at the bottom of the back of the ear to relieve pain
- Aromatherapy: put a drop of lavender on cotton and put it in the ear; use a chamomile tea bag that has been infused for a few minutes and place it on the side of the face or over the ear while it is still warm
- Craniosacral manipulation
- Herbs: warm mullein oil drops in ear
- Homeopathy: pulsatilla, belladonna, or aconite—1 tablet every 4 hours for 2–3 days
- Reflexology: work all fingers and toes paying close attention to the webs between the fingers and toes, especially between the 3rd, 4th, and 5th digits

Emotional Distress

- Aromatherapy: chamomile, frankincense (deepens breathing to induce calmness), marjoram
- Breathing exercises
- Gratitude exercises
- Positive affirmations

Energy Imbalance

- Applied Kinesiology
- Healing Touch
- Magnets
- Polarity Therapy
- Pressure point therapies
- Reiki
- Shiatsu massage
- Thai massage
- Therapeutic Touch

Fatigue

- Aromatherapy: peppermint, rose, rosemary, and basil stimulate the brain; lemon grass and rosemary are best for physical fatigue; use these oils in the bath, in massage oils, in vaporizers, or on a handkerchief; do not use peppermint or rosemary at night because they are too stimulating; rosemary should not be used by people with hypertension or epilepsy
- Herbs: ginseng (600 mg daily) especially for people over the age of 40
- Qigong
- Reflexology: a brisk complete foot treatment for more energy or a slow complete foot treatment to induce sleep
- Supplements: zinc, co-enzyme Q
- Yoga: start with relaxation and gentle movements on your back, progressing to kneeling, standing, and/or seated postures

Feet (Tired)

- Aromatherapy: foot bath of 2 drops each of rosemary, sage, and peppermint oils in basin of hot water; soak for at least 15 minutes; rosemary (20 drops), sage (15 drops), and peppermint (10 drops) mixed in oil base can be applied directly to feet
- Massage
- Reflexology

Fever

- Aromatherapy: tea tree and juniper encourage the body to sweat; lavender and peppermint are cooling; chamomile is soothing and calming; use either in a bath or in cool water to sponge the body
- Herbs: to a large mug of boiling water add juice of 1 lemon, 2 tsp. honey, 1 tsp. grated ginger, 1/2 tsp. cinnamon, 1/2 tsp. nutmeg, and 1 tbsp. brandy or whisky
- Homeopathy: belladonna, aconite, ferrum phosphoricum, gelsemium—1 tablet every 30 minutes for six doses, then every 4 hours—maximum 3 days

Fibromyalgia

- Acupuncture
- Biofeedback
- Herbs: topical capsaicin
- Magnets: sleep on a magnetic mattress and use a magnetic pillow; magnets can also be placed over painful areas during the day
- Supplements: magnesium, malic acid

Fluid Retention

- Massage feet and ankles
- Elevate legs

Headache (Tension)

- Acupressure: press pressure points between eyebrows or at bottom of web between thumb and first finger
- Alexander Technique: helps improve posture to avoid buildup of tension in neck and shoulders
- Aromatherapy: basil, chamomile, massage lavender, peppermint, or eucalyptus around temples; rose compress to eyes
- Chiropractic manipulation
- Herbs: 1/2 tsp. each of betony and skullcap made into tea; ginseng (200 mg daily)

- Homeopathy: bryonia (wild hops), windflower, yellow jasmine, nux vomica—1 tablet every 4 hours as needed—maximum 6 doses
- Pulsating electromagnetic fields
- Relaxation techniques
- Therapeutic Touch
- Yoga

Heart Disease

- Animal-assisted therapy
- Biofeedback
- Chelation therapy
- Herbs: 1–2 capsules of hawthorn four times a day for mild angina
- Meditation
- Supplements: vitamin E, L-carnitine (1,000 mg two times a day); co-enzyme Q (30–100 mg per day) to improve utilization of oxygen at cellular level

Heat Rash

- Herbs: sprinkle arrowroot powder on affected area; 1/2 cup of freshly grated ginger into a quart of boiling water—remove from heat immediately and steep for 5 minutes—cool and sponge ginger water onto affected areas and let it dry

Hemorrhoids

- Aromatherapy: massage geranium, chamomile, or lavender oil, mixed with a carrier oil, into the rectal area as needed
- Herbs: apply aloe vera gel to relieve itching; use compresses of witch hazel to clean area after bowel movement
- Homeopathy: aesculus, aloe, or hamamelis—1 tablet 2 times daily—maximum 2 weeks
- Hydrotherapy: sit in warm bath for 15 minutes several times a day

Hypertension

- Animal-assisted therapy
- Aromatherapy: ylang-ylang, clary sage, lavender, marjoram
- Biofeedback
- Herbs: garlic, hawthorn
- Massage
- Meditation
- Qigong
- Supplements: vitamin C; calcium for pregnancy-induced hypertension
- T'ai Chi
- Yoga

Immune Enhancement

- Aromatherapy: elemi, eucalyptus
- Herbs: echinacea
- Massage
- Qigong
- Supplements: vitamin E, vitamin C, beta-carotene, garlic

Indigestion

- Aromatherapy: basil, chamomile, coriander, ginger, peppermint—use as a tea or in massage oil or warm compress over stomach area
- Herbs: chamomile, peppermint, ginger as a tea; for heaviness after a meal chew on cardamom or fennel seeds
- Homeopathy: windflower; nux vomica—1 tablet hourly for six doses, then three times daily—maximum 1 week

Infection (Bacterial)

- Aromatherapy: calendula, geranium, rosemary, tea tree, lavender, eucalyptus, thyme, niaouli, bergamot—these oils work by attacking the organisms themselves, by killing airborne germs, and by strengthening the immune system

▓ Herbs: echinacea (600 mg three times a day) at first sign of infection; echinacea may be combined with goldenseal; garlic (2 g daily) in capsules

Infection (Fungal)

▓ Aromatherapy: calendula, lemon balm, rosemary, tea tree

▓ Herbs: garlic

Infection (Viral)

▓ Aromatherapy: eucalyptus, lemon balm, tea tree

▓ Herbs: goldenseal, echinacea, garlic

▓ Supplements: zinc, selenium

Infertility

▓ Meditation for unexplained infertility

▓ Supplements: zinc for men

Inflammation

▓ Aromatherapy: benzoin, birch, chamomile, clary sage, elemi, fennel, geranium, helichrysum, jasmine, myrrh, patchouli, rose, sandalwood

▓ Bee venom may slow down the body's inflammatory response by inhibiting the amount of free radicals or by stimulating the adrenal glands to release cortisol

▓ Homeopathy: belladonna

▓ Hydrotherapy: applications of heat and cold

▓ Magnets

Insomnia

▓ Aromatherapy: chamomile, which can also be used with children; clary sage, lavender, marjoram, neroli, or vetiver in bath or a pillow or as a room fragrance

- Exercise: not later than early evening
- Herbs: valerian, lemon balm, catnip, hops, passion flower, skullcap teas (if taste is unpleasant, add sugar, honey, or lemon)
- Homeopathy: windflower, nux vomica, arsenicum album—1 tablet before bed for 10 days or until improved
- Hydrotherapy: warm baths
- Magnets: use magnetic pillow or pad for sedating effect
- Meditation

Jet Lag

- Herbs: melatonin
- Drink fluids and avoid alcohol; do in-flight stretches

Labor Pain

- Aromatherapy: blend of clary sage, rose, and ylang-ylang for massage—deep massage of lower back and hips during contractions, between contractions massage shoulders, back, hands, and feet; if contractions are lagging, a light massage of the breasts may stimulate activity
- Herbs: red raspberry tea, black cohosh tea
- Hypnosis

Liver Disease

- Herbs: milk thistle, dandelion root tea
- Hydrotherapy: take steam baths or saunas frequently to help body eliminate toxins

Memory Loss

- Aromatherapy: basil, black pepper, coriander, ginger, rosemary, thyme
- Exercise
- Herbs: 2 capsules twice a day of ginkgo
- Supplements: vitamin B6

Menopause

- Aromatherapy: geranium, rose, fennel in bath or in body creams
- Herbs: black cohosh (4 tablets daily), vitex, agnue castii, rehmannia, ginseng, wild yam as tea; Chinese tonic of He Shou Wu, dong quai
- Meditation
- Supplements: vitamin E (200–800 IU daily), soy protein (50 g daily)

Menstrual Discomfort

- Aromatherapy: basil; clary sage massage or warm compress; massage abdomen and lower back with jasmine, marjoram
- Herbs: tea of agnus castus with rosemary for premenstrual water retention; black haw for cramps—4 tsp. in glass of warm water, repeat after 4 hours if necessary; Chinese tonic of dong quai
- Homeopathy: viburnum, magnesium phosphate, sepia—1 tablet every 2–4 hours—maximum 12 doses
- Hydrotherapy: warm compresses
- Reflexology: massage uterine reflexes below inside ankle bones and ovarian reflexes beneath outside ankle bones
- Supplements: calcium and manganese, fish oil, parsley, celery, and dandelion leaves are all mild diuretics
- Yoga stretches and more relaxation and breathing exercises

Migraine Headaches

- Aromatherapy: green apple (inhalant), lavender, mellissa, or peppermint put on a facecloth with cool water and used as a compress on the forehead or back of the neck
- Biofeedback
- Herbs: feverfew (prophylaxis)
- Homeopathy: iris, sanguinaria, glonoine—1 tablet every 30 minutes until improved—maximum 6 doses
- Hypnosis
- Pressure-point therapies
- Pulsating electromagnetic fields

Morning Sickness

- Acupressure: wristband—small weights that exerts pressure on a specific pressure point on the wrist
- Herbs: peppermint, catnip, ginger, chamomile teas

Muscle Soreness

- Aromatherapy: chamomile, juniper
- Herbs: rub in wintergreen oil or capsicum cream
- Hydrotherapy: spa
- Massage
- Yoga

Nausea

- Acupressure: wristband—small weights that exert pressure on a specific pressure point on the wrist
- Aromatherapy: ginger, lavender, peppermint used as a compress and as teas
- Healing Touch
- Homeopathy: ipecacuanha, sepia, clossypium—1 tablet every half-hour—maximum 12 doses
- Imagery
- Reiki
- Therapeutic Touch

Osteoarthritis

- Acupuncture
- Alexander Technique: to relieve muscular tension and uneven weight-bearing
- Bioelectromagnetics
- Herbs: glucosamine and chondroitin to help restore joint integrity; natural anti-inflammatories like willowbark, turmeric, and ginger
- Hydrotherapy: soak in hot water or spa frequently; use ice packs on inflamed joints
- Pressure point therapies

- Relaxation exercises
- Supplements: vitamin B6 (100 mg two times a day)
- Yoga: practice slowly, seeing how far you can move affected joints without pain; do not exercise when joints are inflamed

Osteoporosis

- Exercise: weight bearing unless advanced stage of disease
- Herbs: a tea of stinging nettles, alfalfa, or sage
- Supplements: calcium, vitamins D and C, hormone replacement therapy

Pain

- Alexander Technique
- Chiropractic manipulation
- Healing Touch
- Herbs: feverfew
- Hydrotherapy: hot water packs
- Hypnosis
- Imagery
- Magnets
- Pressure-point therapies
- Reiki
- Sports massage
- Therapeutic Touch
- Trager Approach
- Trigger-point massage

Poison Ivy and Poison Oak

- Rinse the exposed area with soap and cold water; mix baking soda with water to form a paste and apply it to skin; once the paste has hardened, remove with cool water and apply a thin layer of honey to the area.
- For itching and discomfort, grind 1 cup raw, whole oats to a fine powder and add to tepid bath—soak for 20–30 minutes

Premenstrual Syndrome

- Acupuncture
- Aromatherapy: massage or warm bath with rose oil, clary sage, ylang-ylang, lavender, lemon grass, sandalwood, jasmine, bergamot—you will have to decide, by trial and error, which one of these oils best suits you
- Deep breathing exercises for a least 20 minutes a day
- Herbs: vitex, black cohosh extract, agnus-castus (10–20 drops each morning); Helonias; Chinese tonic of dong quai
- Homeopathy: windflower, pulsatilla, lachesis—1 tablet two times daily—maximum 1 week; may be repeated next period
- Meditation
- Reflexology: massage uterine reflexes below inside ankle bones and ovarian reflexes beneath outside ankle bones
- Supplements: vitamin B6, 2–3 g capsule of combined fish oil and evening primrose oil

Prostate Enlargement (Benign)

- Herbs: Saw palmetto (160 mg two times a day) pygeum africanum, stinging nettle root tea
- Supplements: 30 mg of zinc picolinate daily; add soy foods to diet

Psoriasis

- Diet: include foods with zinc, beta-carotene, vitamin D, and omega-3 fatty acids; avoid liver and other organ meats, foods that aggravate psoriasis
- Herbs: aloe vera extract in topical application—apply three times a day—do not cover
- Homeopathy: sepai, arsenicum iodatum, petroleum—1 tablet two times daily—maximum 2 weeks
- Sunshine on the skin is helpful

Sciatica

- Acupuncture
- Applied Kinesiology
- Chiropractic manipulation
- Hydrotherapy: warm water jets
- Reflexology

Sexual Dysfunction

- Herbs: ginkgo (180 to 240 mg daily) for erectile problems; ashwaganda
- Hypnotherapy and imagery

Shingles

- Aromatherapy: eucalyptus, tea tree, lavender, chamomile, bergamot—smooth the oil gently over the affected areas and down either side of the spine; if body is too painful to touch, add oils to a water spray or use in a bath
- Herbs: echinacea (up to 2 g daily); St. John's wort tea, aloe vera gel to blistering area

Sinus Problems

- Aromatherapy: basil, marjoram or eucalyptus—put on handkerchief or use with a vaporizer
- Herbs: ephedra, goldenseal, yarrow, coltsfoot—make a tea using 2 tsp. of herb per cup; use herbs in cream or oil and massage the sinus areas
- Homeopathy: hydrastis, kali bichromicum—1 tablet three times daily—maximum 10 days
- Hydrotherapy: hot and cold compresses, steam inhalation, nasal lavage
- Reflexology: massage the sinus reflexes on the tips of the fingers and toes

Skin (Dry)

- Aromatherapy: mix 2 drops each of sandalwood, rose, and geranium oil with a tablespoon of almond oil—use as a topical evening moisturizer; other oils good for dry skin include jasmine, orange, and ylang-ylang used in a moisturizer or in a bath

Sore Throat

- Aromatherapy: several drops of sandalwood on handkerchief or mix with carrier oil and massage into throat area and then wrap something warm around the throat
- Herbs: mix 1 cup of warm water with 1/4 teaspoon of salt and 1/2 teaspoon of goldenseal powder
- Homeopathy: monkshood, poison ivy, belladonna—1 tablet every 2 hours for 6 doses, then every 4 hours—maximum 3 days
- Reflexology: massage the throat reflexes around the "neck" of the big toes and thumbs

Sprain and Strains

- Aromatherapy: chamomile, ginger, lavender as massage to area
- Healing Touch
- Herbs: 1/4 cup each of dry mustard powder and flour with warm water to make a thick paste, spread the paste onto cheesecloth or gauze, roll it up, and apply to the strained area
- Homeopathy: poison ivy—1 tablet three times daily—maximum 2 weeks
- Hydrotherapy: cold compresses to reduce swelling first 24 hours; then warm compresses to increase circulation
- Magnets: cover area with magnetic pad and secure with an Ace bandage—12 hours on and 12 hours off
- Myofascial release
- Pressure-point therapies
- Reiki
- Therapeutic Touch

Surgery

- Hypnotherapy and visualization before surgery
- Magnets: place magnets over the incision site for 24 to 48 hours before surgery to improve postoperative recovery, place magnets over wound after surgery
- Meditation before and after surgery

Stress

- Aromatherapy: juniper, lavender, vetiver, ylang ylang, jasmine—use in massage oil or put in bath
- Breathing exercises; alternate nostril breathing (pranayama)
- Exercise
- Meditation
- Yoga: focus on slow movements and long exhalations

Sunburn

- Herbs: soak a soft cloth in cooled black or green tea and spread over the burned area—leave on 15–30 minutes; apply aloe vera sap to area
- Hydrotherapy: soak in a bath of tepid water and baking soda (1 pound) for 20–30 minutes; later that day or next take a tepid bath with 1 or 2 cups of milk added
- Grated potato applied directly to the skin will decrease pain and prevent blistering; wrap in place with a clean cloth

Tension

- Aromatherapy: hot bath or massage using one of the following oils—bergamot, rose, cedarwood, chamomile, geranium, lavender, melissa, orange, or sandalwood
- Feldenkrais Method
- Healing Touch
- Herbs: valerian, passion flower, kava kava, ginseng as teas

- Massage
- Meditation
- Reiki
- Therapeutic Touch

Tinnitus

- Supplements: vitamin B12

Urinary Tract Infection

- Aromatherapy: bergamot, sandalwood, lavender, or juniper in bath water
- Herbs: 2 capsules three times a day of uva ursi until symptoms disappear
- Supplements: unsweetened cranberry juice (300 ml daily) and vitamin C
- Urinate after sexual activity
- Drink plenty of water

Warts

- Aromatherapy: 1 drop each of lemon, thyme, and tea tree oil mixed in a base oil and swabbed two times a day
- Hypnosis
- Imagery

Weight Control

- Aromatherapy: green apple
- Exercise
- Herbs: evening primrose oil
- Supplements: 2.5 g of vitamin B5, four times a day

Wounds

- Aromatherapy: to disinfect—bergamot, chamomile, clary sage, jasmine, juniper, lavender, rose, tea tree; to relieve pain—bergamot, chamomile, geranium, jasmine, lavender, rosemary; to stop bleeding—cypress, geranium, rose; to reduce inflammation—chamomile, geranium, helichrysum, jasmine, patchouli; to promote formation of scar tissue—bergamot, chamomile, helichrysum, jasmine

- Bioelectromagnetics

- Herbs: echinacea, goldenseal

- Hydrotherapy: warm water irrigation

Index

ASCH (American Society of Clinical Hypnosis), 217

Aserinsky, Eugene, 229

assessments (chiropractic diagnostic methods), 135

asthi, 55

asthma, alternative therapies, 320-321

astragalus, TCM (Traditional Chinese Medicine) treatments, 45

astral body layer (auric fields), 26

athlete's foot, alternative therapies, 321

attention (meditation), 203

Auckett, Amelia, 142

auras, 22, 26-27. *See also* chakras

auscultation/olfaction (TCM diagnostic methods), 42

autonomic nervous system (biofeedback), 242

awareness through movement (Feldenkrais Method), 252

Ayurveda, 51
  Adhibhautika diseases, 56
  Adhidaivika diseases, 56
  Adhyatmika diseases, 56
  composite body types, 54-55
  dhatus, 55
  diagnostic methods, 57
  doshas, 53, 56-60, 64-67
  five elements of, 52
  goal of, 52
  malas, 55
  marma therapy, 63
  prana, 55
  pranayama, 62
  treatments, 58-64

B

baby massage, 142, 150, 153

back pain, alternative therapies, 321-322

bacterial infection, alternative therapies, 332

balance
  circadian rhythms, 18
  musical rhythms, 18-19
  problems, alternative therapies, 322

balancing doshas, 56-57, 66-67

basil (aromatherapy), 124

baths, 296, 301

BCIA (Biofeedback Certification Institute of America), 242

Beardell, Alan G., 178

bee stings, alternative therapies, 322

"being attacked" nightmares, 235

"being chased" nightmares, 235

"being unprepared for an exam" nightmares, 235

Beings of Light, 20

belladonna (deadly nightshade), homeopathy, 113

BEM (Bioelectromagnetics)
  broken bones, 323
  crystal cards, 289
  crystal composition, 284
  crystal meditation, 291
  crystal resonance, 287
  crystal selection, 290
  development of, 284
  electrocrystal therapy, 289
  electroencephalography, 288
  electromyography, 288
  electronic gem therapy, 289
  electroretinography, 288
  endogenous magnetic fields, 286-287
  exogenous magnetic fields, 287
  gemstones, 285
  geomagnetic fields, 285
  headaches, 331, 335
  low energy emission therapy, 288
  "magnetic field deficiency syndrome", 284
  magnetic therapies, 288-289, 292-293
  migraine headaches, 335
  neuromagnetic stimulation, 288
  osteoarthritis, 336
  Pink Bubble guided imagery, 291-292
  resonance, 287
  sleep, 286
  sprains/strains, 340
  surgery, 341
  TCES (transcranial electrostimulation), 288
  TENS (transcultaneous electrical nerve stimulation), 288
  tension headaches, 331
  wounds, 343

bergamot (aromatherapy), 124

Bhakti Yoga, goals of, 190

bian zheng, 41

Bioelectromagnetics. *See* BEM (Bioelectromagnetics)

"bioenergy", 22

biofeedback, 245
  ADD (Attention Deficit Disorder), 321
  anxiety, 319
  asthma, 320
  autonomic nervous system, 242
  back pain, 321
  cardiovascular, 243
  certification, 242
  circulation (poor), 325

frequencies, 24
functions of, 23-24
gemstones, 290
hand chakras, 23
heart chakras, 24-25
navel chakras. *See* sexual chakras
root chakras, characteristics of, 24
sexual chakras, characteristics of, 24
solar plexus chakras, 24, 28
third eye chakras, characteristics of, 25
throat chakras, characteristics of, 25

chamomile
aromatherapy, 124
herbal medicine, 90, 93

chanting (Native American medicine), 75

chaos theory, 108

Chelation Therapies
EDTA (ethylene diamine tetraacetic acid), 298-299
heart disease, 331

chest congestion, alternative therapies, 324

chi, 22, 37, 40. *See also* prana; qi
Five Phases Theory, 38
meridians, 27
movement therapies, 248
Qigong, 249-250, 253-256
T'ai Chi, 249-256
tan diens, 28
tan t'ien, 255

children, AAT (Animal-Assisted Therapy), 305

Chinese compasses, 39

Chinese medicine. *See* TCM (Traditional Chinese Medicine)

chiropractic therapies
back pain, 322
carpal tunnel syndrome, 324

common ailments, 138
development of, 132
diagnostic methods, 135-136
education, 132
headaches (tension), 330
hypermobile spinal joins, 136
pain management, 337
palpation, 136
philosophies of, 133-135
sacroiliac joints, 133
sciatica, 339
SMT (spinal manual therapy), 136
spinal vertebrae, 133
treatments, 137-138
vertebral subluxation, 132, 135

chloresterol (high), alternative therapies, 325

chondroitin, herbal medicine, 90

circadian rhythms, 18

circles, significance of in Native American medicine, 71

circulation (poor), alternative therapies, 325

clary sage (aromatherapy), 124

cold sores, alternative therapies, 326

colds, alternative therapies, 325

colic, alternative therapies, 326

Collinge, William, 170

colloquial prayer (religious healing), 277

colonics, 297-298

combined manual therapies
Applied Kinesiology, 177-183
exercise, 184
meridians, 183
neurolymphatic points, 179, 183

neurovascular points, 179-181
nutrition, 183-184
Polarity Therapy, 177-183
stress relief exercises, 184

comfrey, herbal medicine, 93

common colds, alternative therapies, 325

companion animals, 303
AAT (Animal-Assisted Therapy) registration, 304
AIDS, 311
benefits of, 306
children, 305
grooming/maintenance, 311
handler certification, 305
handler training, 305
hippotherapy, 308
HIV, 311
hygiene, 312
long-term health care facilities, 307-309
obedience training, 304
pet interaction, 312
pet visits, 308
resident animal, 309
service dogs, 310
temperment, 304
veterinary care, 311

compasses (Chinese), 39

compassion, energy-balancing therapies, 170

complementary medicine, defining, 6

composite body types (Ayurveda), 54-55

compresses
as detoxifying therapy, 300
hydrotherapy, 296

concentration (meditation), 203

confession and absolution (religious healing remedies), 274

congestion (chest), alternative therapies, 324